It's All in My Head!

It's All in My Head!
A story about hearing voices

Written and illustrated by:
Mick Deschrijver

Translated with the help of:
Nicole Schnackenberg

Copyright © Mick Deschrijver 2018

All rights reserved. No part of this publication may be reproduced or transmitted in any form or by any means, electronic or mechanical including photocopying, recording or any information storage or retrieval system, without prior permission in writing from the publishers.

The right of Mick Deschrijver to be identified as the author of this work has been asserted by him in accordance with the Copyright, Designs and Patents Act 1988

First published in the United Kingdom in 2018 by
The Choir Press

ISBN: 978-1-911589-56-3

Cover: Mick Deschrijver (program 'Sketches')
Illustrations: Mick Deschrijver (program 'Sketches')
Translation: Mick and Nicole Schnackenberg
Foreword: D. Corstens, psychiatrist
Website: http://www.itsallinmyhead.eu
To contact Mick: mickdeschrijver@gmail.com

Foreword

'My voice will go with you…' is the title of a book by Milton H. Erickson (1901-1980), who is often referred to as an 'American healer'. If I hadn't known that title I would have been even more shocked when Mick told me that he heard a voice which had my name. "This is because you don't respect professional boundaries. You make yourself too important. You use your patients to gratify your own narcissism. You need their dependency…" These were the accusations a voice within me uttered.

I almost pissed my pants when I saw how Mick had portrayed 'my voice'! *A wolf in sheep's clothing!* Mick really knows me, I thought. He knows that I am a human being behind the role in the consulting room. "That you can lie, that you can also be mean, that you don't know sometimes, that you do things without thinking, a stupid sheep. But also that you want sincerely to help and don't give up easily. That you have really helped…" These were the other voices I heard. I was also proud when I saw the drawing…and touched by its profundity and the message it contained. I now know for sure that the Dirk voice is supportive towards Mick, and does not tell fairy tales.

I am proud of Mick that he has accomplished so much and proud of myself that I played a role in his road to recovery. I am proud that I eventually took another road in my journey. That's the way it goes with travellers.

I can envisage us sitting on the first floor of the Crisis Centre. A dark evening with special lighting in the room with a sloping floor. No artificial light. Mick was sitting opposite me, with his back against the wall. He wanted to die. Period. I had talked to the voice of someone else only once before. I wasn't convinced that the protocol would have a solution in this instance. But I couldn't see another option. In some way or another we were 'carried'. It was all or nothing. It went well, like with the other voice hearer, with whom Mick became friends some time later. 'De Brutaalste'* became an ally. The beginning of a road to recovery. The voices as guides on this journey without a goal.

Many people contributed to Mick's recovery. I especially want to mention the workers of the Crisis Centre and the local psychiatric hospital, even though Mick didn't always agree on the way you did your job and could really complain and moan about it. These workers, in spite of everything, supported Mick and myself even when we didn't know how to proceed in terms of Mick's care. They admitted Mick as an inpatient, again and again, without any further questions asked.

Without their support and trust this book would not have been written. And thanks also, of course, to Emilia who successfully challenged Mick to let go the role of psychiatric patient. And to the students who listened breathlessly to Mick when he told them about his voices.
Mick transformed his hardship into resources, into a polyphony. This book is a witness of that. This is a book of hope. A book of humanity. I recommend it to every human being, that means to every voice hearer.

His voices will go with you...
Dirk Corstens,
Maastricht

* *one of the voices.*

Introduction

My name is Mick and I'm forty-one years old. I'm single and I live together with my stuffed toy animals in my cosy apartment in the south of the Netherlands. I have many hobbies and some friends. I play sports every once in awhile and I also work every now and again. Very normal, just like anyone else.

But there is something different, something that's outside of many people's usual experience. I hear voices that other people cannot hear.

I have been hearing voices my whole life. I don't know any different, it has always been like this. Very often when I tell people about this for the first time, they respond with things like: how horrible, how terrible, how bad this must be for you. And although it's definitely not always a bed of roses and has been very difficult in the past, nowadays this kind of reaction makes me very sad.

There's also a second kind of response: the assumption that I am a 'schizophrenic'. This is due to the fact that I hear voices that no other person can hear. I do understand that people who have never heard voices themselves, or who do hear voices and are very afraid of them, don't know any better and need, or want, to see this as a form of illness. But it isn't that simple to me and I have a different view on it. I personally don't believe that hearing voices is an illness or a sign of illness. But I do think that it can make you very ill if you don't learn how to cope with it.

There was a period when I didn't know how to cope with the voices myself. It felt like I didn't have a life: the voices were my life. They determined what I did, or did not do, what I said, or did not say, and what I thought, or did not think. It felt like there was no 'me' anymore. I was terrified of the voices. Given the choice, I would have wanted to get rid of them, the sooner the better. I never took the effort to really listen to them, to actively hear what they really had to tell me. I was way too afraid of them. I was just shouting and cursing at them so they would leave me alone, but they did not.

Now, many years later, I have learned to really listen to the voices. And it turns out that they have really useful things to say. By listening to them, and to their story, and by asking the right questions, I now know what my own story is. I now know who I am.

These days I'm really grateful for my voices. They (together with other things) have made me the person I am today. I still learn something new from them every day. They keep me alert and they point out the things and issues I still need to work on. They have saved my life, over and over again, sometimes literally.

So, voices aren't always horrible, terrible, bad, or negative. They also are a gift, something to be grateful for. That's why I want to explain some things about my voices to you, about their background and their role in my life. In other words, I want to tell you their story!

I now experience my voices as helpers who are sometimes very clumsy with their choice of words, or speak in some kind of code language. For many years I have seen it as my duty to act like some kind of detective to crack the code. When you have cracked that code, there is a lot of useful and important information to discover!

Why do I want to write this book and to share my experiences with you?

I would like to show the world that hearing voices is not an illness in and of itself, but that it can make you very ill if you don't learn how to cope with it.

Within the mental health system, professionals too often assume that voices do not make any sense. They typically assume that they have nothing to do with the person and that they kind of come out of the blue. Very frequently, professionals don't look beyond voices as a symptom of a supposed illness. It's really rare for people to be asked: "What happened to you? What is your story?" ...even though, in my opinion, these are the most important questions!

With this book I want to make it clear that voices do not come out of the blue. They make sense and give very important information about the person and their life. They should not be made to disappear, and they should not be silenced (for example with medication). They should be really listened to. Voices are there for a reason: they have important information and are usually more like allies than enemies! (I'm not saying that you should quit taking your medication by the way. If that is something you would like to do, you should always talk to your doctor! Or find a doctor who is willing to help you with this).

What should you expect from this book?

One of my voices, Rik, loves to draw. Thanks to him, I discovered that I liked drawing myself as well, but not so much on paper, but rather on my iPad.

One day, the thought came to my mind to draw my voices so that I could tell their story. After drawing some of them, I realised that I could not include their whole story inside one drawing. And that's how the idea of this book came to life.

The drawings will be the starting point. I will use them to introduce my voices to you. I will tell you some things about their character, their role in my life, when they came, what was happening in my life at that point, and how they tried to help me. Maybe this will help you to see what I mean when I say that voices are not always horrible, terrible etc. That they are a logical response to what is happening in your life.

The drawings contained in this book are made with the program 'Sketches' on the iPad. Usually, I used an image I found on the internet as the basis of the drawing and I went on to adjust, change, and combine it until it looked like what I needed. I think this is important to mention, at least.

Another important thing to mention is that I am Dutch and most of the names of my voices are Dutch. It doesn't feel very respectful to change/translate their names. I discussed this with the voices and it's something they really don't want, so I will respect that. At some points, I make some exceptions, to make this book easier to read. In all the other cases I will explain (if necessary) what every name means. I hope this won't bother you.

I hope you will enjoy reading this book.

Mick.

De Lieve Vrouwenstem
('The Voice of the Sweet Old Lady')

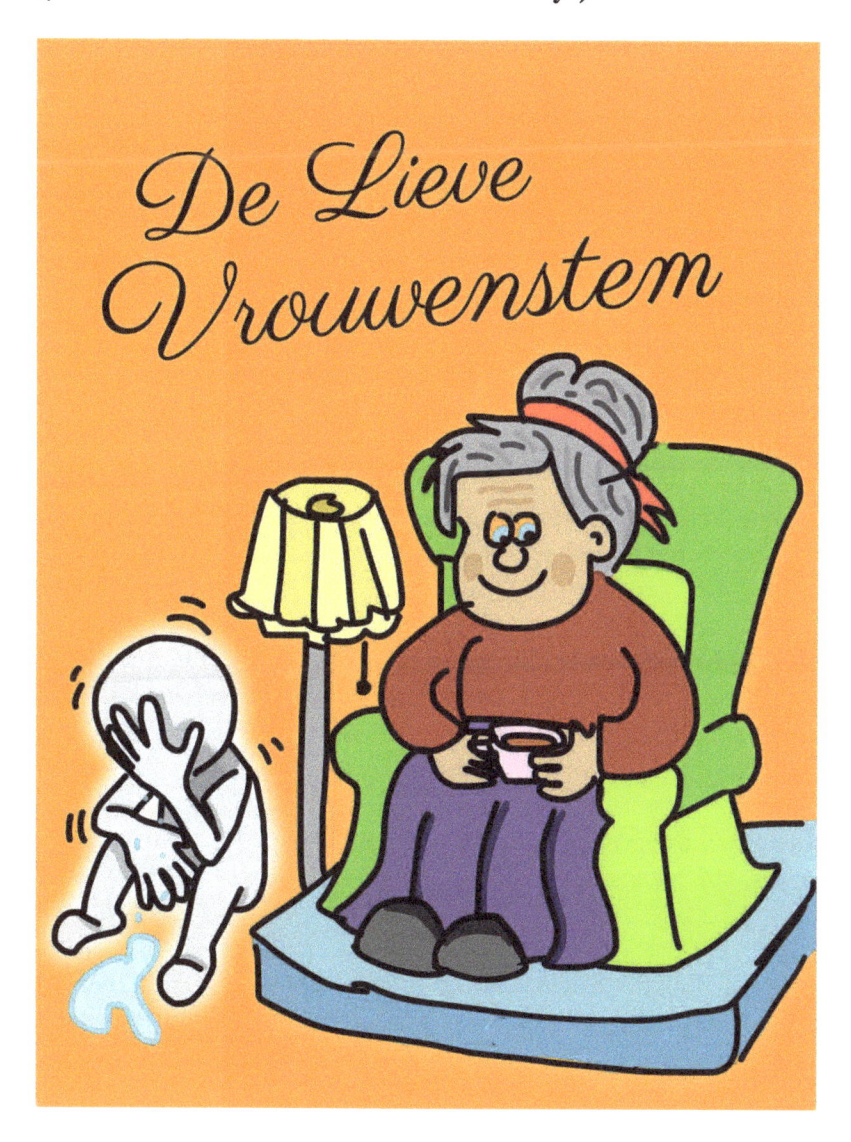

When I was nineteen years old my Granny died. To me this felt like the end of the world. Granny was my buddy and she was probably the only person on earth that I completely trusted.

When I was born, my Mother could not take care of me. She did take care of my older brother, but she ignored me completely.

As my Father had a very busy job and was also very active in all kind of committees and stuff, he was away most of the time. Therefore, my Granny came to our house from Monday until Friday to take care of me and my older brother.

This meant that each Monday morning she had to cross half of the country to get to us. She then travelled back each Friday evening. During this time, she left my Grandpa at home alone.

My Granny kept doing this for about three years. At that point my Grandpa got really ill and she needed to stay at home to take care of him.

My best and happiest early childhood memories are of the times when Granny came to visit us. She usually brought her brother along and we all played a lot of games. The two of them were incredible game-fanatics. These are very precious memories to me.

I also went to sleepovers at my Granny's house a lot. During these sleepovers, she took me to her weekly card night where I was spoilt rotten!

One of the highlights for me during these sleepovers at my Granny's place was a simple cup of leek soup. Just instant, leek soup. But, oh, it was heavenly to me!

Sometimes, Granny took me shopping and we went to a 'posh' store where I could pick something out for myself. I remember a plastic football I once got and a very funny pair of pyjamas with a happy bear on them. Simple things, but they meant the world to me. Just for a very short moment while I was with her, I felt like a normal kid. Everything was quiet, everything was safe, and I didn't have to keep my guard up all the time.

Granny was my 'safe person' and also my safe haven. If too much shit was going on at home I ran away to Granny's house, on the other side of the country. Granny almost always brought me back to my parents immediately, in an attempt to avoid more trouble for me.

Later on, my Granny got sick. That was in my final year of High School. I remember it so well. I remember going to visit her in the hospital. The doctors told her there was nothing else that could be done for her. I saw her lying in the bed: my always so funny and happy Granny, full of laughing wrinkles. Now she was lying in her bed crying and very skinny.

I brought Granny a card with a yellow inflatable animal inside and the text 'Get Well Soon' on its stomach. I looked at her and asked her very quietly: "It's not going very well, is it Granny?". She looked at me, shook her head and started to cry again. I felt tormented inside.

Granny didn't want to die in the hospital, so she went back home to her apartment. Every day after school I took the train and travelled for two hours to get to her house. I sat at her bedside, fetched some groceries for her, went to bed, and the next morning I took the first train back home to go to school. I never once thought of not doing this for her. Granny had always been there for me. Now it was my turn to be there for, and with, her.

About two weeks before my final exams started, Granny was doing so badly that she asked for a priest to come and administer the Last Rites to her. The whole family were present. The priest was sitting at the end of her bed. My Granny would not be my Granny if she couldn't make a joke at this point. So, she insisted on telling the priest a final joke. She hardly had the energy to tell it. She even threw up whilst telling it, but this was what she wanted to do. That was my Granny!

After the Last Rites, we all came to her bed, one by one, to say our farewells to her. By the time it was my turn, Granny was really weak. She had been given a lot of Morphine. Granny grabbed my hand, squeezed it so hard that it hurt, and whispered in my ear: "It's not your fault. You are perfect the way you are, don't you ever forget that!". All the while she kept squeezing my hand even more and it really hurt!

For many years I have asked myself whether this powerful hand squeeze was especially for me, or if it was the result of the Morphine. I have never got the true answer to my question.

At the end of this day we went back home. Because my final exams were underway, I could not go to visit her every day anymore.

Granny died a week before my first final exam. I felt so incredibly sad, and also very guilty. I had been going to visit her for all that time, but at the moment she might have needed me the most, the very last moment of her life, I wasn't with her. I still find that very difficult. It feels like I betrayed her.

On the same day my Granny died, or maybe the next day, I started to hear a very friendly voice of an old lady. It wasn't the same sound as the voice of my Granny, but she did have the same kind of jokes and the same soothing tone. It sounded so calming and soothing that it didn't frighten me. On the contrary, I actually really liked it. At first I didn't even notice that I was hearing a voice. To me it was absolutely normal.

I gave this voice a descriptive name: 'De Lieve Vrouwenstem', 'The Voice of the Sweet Old Lady', because that's what she was: sweet. She was actually around all of the time. She didn't always speak to me but I could sense her presence. Mainly, she came when I was feeling sad or lonely and could use some comfort or support.

Just by hearing her quiet, calm and soothing voice, I would feel a bit better. The things she said to me were almost always the same: "You are perfect the way you are", "It is not your fault, there was nothing you could do about it", "It has nothing to do with you". Always the same sentences, or with a slight variation on these sentences. But that didn't really matter to me. Every time I heard her voice it had the same calming influence on me.

Over the years, 'De Lieve Vrouwenstem' spoke less and less to me. She was still there, I could feel it, but she didn't necessarily speak to me. I noticed that I could call her if I felt I needed her. I could literally say to her: "Listen, I'm having a hard time. I feel lonely. I need you now" and she would immediately be there with her calm, supportive and soothing words.

As time went on, she did not come on every occasion when I asked her to come. At those moments, I could still feel her presence, but she didn't always speak to me anymore.

I think this had to do with the fact that, over the years, I learned some coping skills. I acquired some tools to calm myself down, to soothe and support myself. So I didn't always need her anymore, even though it sometimes felt like I did.

When 'De Lieve Vrouwenstem' started to 'withdraw' from me, it felt as though she was betraying me and I was on my own again. Yet, over the years I have changed my view and opinion on this. I think she was trying to show me that I was ready to trust myself, to allow me to find out that I had the strength and the skills to cope with situations myself.

Today 'De Lieve Vrouwenstem' is still a presence, but she hardly speaks anymore. Things need to be seriously overwhelming or really bad for her to come and help me. I do miss her sometimes and I wish she was still around, but I try to see it as a compliment that she isn't. Her absence means that she is convinced that I can trust myself, that I have the power and the skills to cope. She believes in me, even in those moments when I can't believe in myself (yet).

During my life, I didn't get as much love and attention from the people around me who were important to me. Instead, I got a lot of indications that the world wasn't a safe place, especially that the people within that world were not to be trusted. No one was to be trusted.

'De Lieve Vrouwenstem' always tried to help me with my lack of self-worth and self-esteem. She also helped me with my lack of experienced love from the people around me. She helped me to see and to experience that I could trust myself, so I didn't need to depend on the trustworthiness of others.

I really do want to emphasise that, even though this voice reminds me a lot of my Granny, she is NOT my Granny. It is a voice that sounds completely different to my Granny's voice, with a different accent, but with the same kind of sound and the same messages that my Granny gave me. But she is not my Granny.

De Brutaalste
('The Most Rude One')

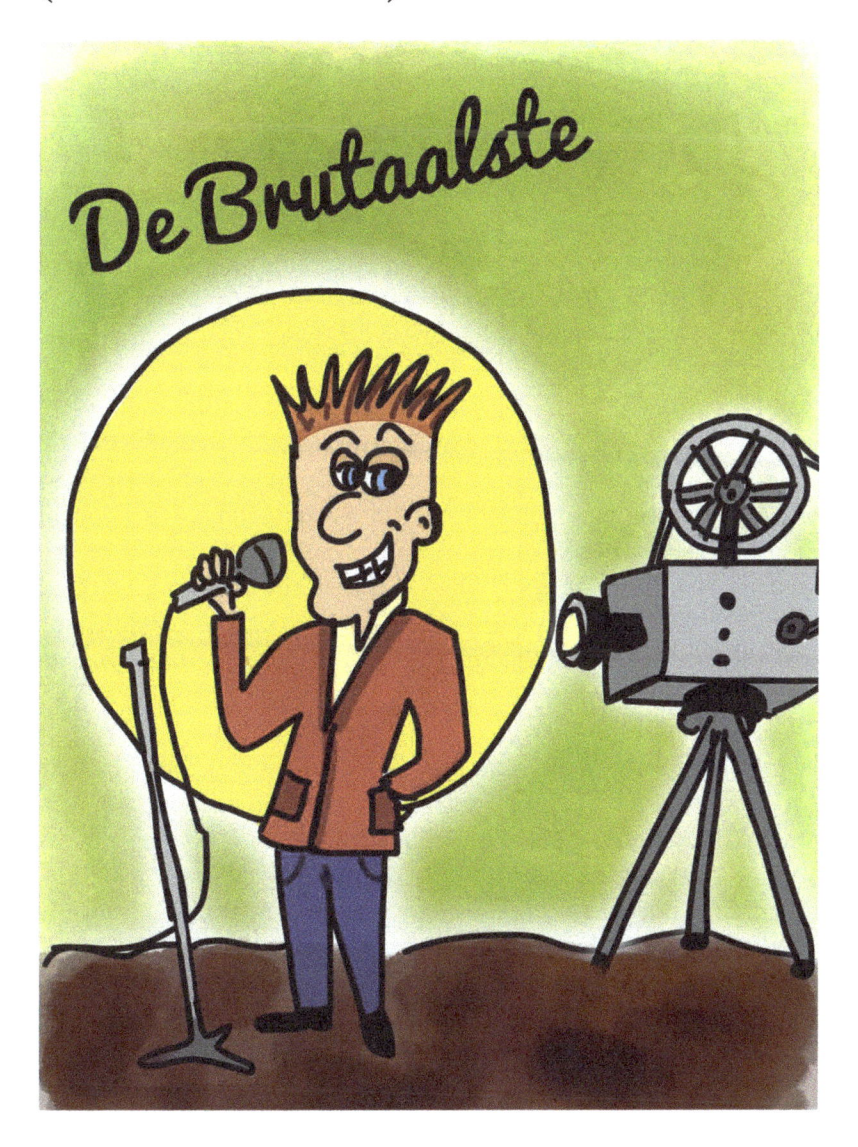

When I was in High School I had no idea what I wanted to do when I grew up. The only thing I really wanted was for my parents, especially my Dad, to be proud of me. That wish was the reason it took me a pretty long time to figure out what I wanted to do with my life. The first thing that came to my mind was a desire to go into the Police Academy. But the main reason I wanted to do this was because it was something my Dad always wanted to do, but couldn't because he didn't get in.

So my next choice was the Sports Academy. This was also a choice based on pleasing my Dad. Although I loved sports, I could not see myself being engaged in sports the whole day long, every day, for the rest of my life.

Deep inside, I did know what I wanted to do: I wanted to help people, especially children who were really struggling in their lives. So I wanted to study to become a care worker for inpatients. It's a course that doesn't exist anymore. It became part of another course (that also doesn't exist anymore). When I shared this desire with my Dad, he laughed in my face. He told me that I was not going to become rich with this job and so I gave up my dream and decided that I had to become a physical therapist.

But as soon as they told me during the Open Day that I had to take anatomy classes, in which we were going to study real (dead, but real) human muscles, I definitely let go of this idea too. Not my cup of tea!

In the end, I decided to do something I wanted to do, to become a care worker in an inpatient unit. I also felt inspired to do this course because I wanted to know what was wrong with me. My whole life I felt different from others but I didn't understand why. So I hoped this course would help me to find the answer to my question.

As this specific course no longer existed, I started to study Social Work. I could have done this in the city where I grew up, the city where my parents were living, but I wanted to be as far away from them as possible. Because I had to subscribe to a new school months before my final exams, I decided to study in a city near to my Granny's home. But by the time I was due to start my course, my Granny had died and I was all alone in this unfamiliar city.

Because Granny died just before my final exams, I didn't do too well and had to retake some of them. Even then, I barely made it - but I made it! I was not able to start looking for housing in my new city due to the fact that I had to retake my exams. I didn't know if I was going to graduate or if I would have to redo the whole year.

By that time, I had become very afraid of people, so I preferred not to live in a dorm with lots of other students. I wanted to find something just for me, with no other people to share things with or, even worse, that I had to talk to. But as I have already said, because of the retake of my exams I was late looking for a room in a city that didn't have too many rooms for their new students. I ended up living in a student house with a total of thirty students. There could not have been a worse nightmare in my eyes!

Anyway, I started my Social Work studies even though I was terrified of people. The studying itself came very easily and naturally to me. I didn't have to do too much. The internships, however, where I had to deal with people, were a lot harder on me.

Living in the student house also felt very scary. The first couple of weeks I went to the kitchen at night to cook, hoping that it would be abandoned and that everyone else would be asleep, so I didn't need to talk to anyone. I locked myself up in my small room and felt completely lost in this huge house.

I went to my parents' house every weekend because I had a weekend job over there. As soon as I finished my working day, I spent the rest of my time with my boyfriend. He was studying in a different city and also came home every weekend to work and to see me.

My Dad still didn't approve of my course. He always asked me when I was going to do a 'real course'. All my enthusiastic stories about the sport, drama, and music lessons I really loved could not be seen as something serious by him. It was very difficult for him that I had chosen a 'lower' kind of education despite the fact that my High School diploma qualified me for university-level study. He (and my Mum also) felt that I was doing something below my level of education. They might have been right about that, but I really did love what I was doing.

Because of my Dad's many derogatory remarks, I decided not to tell my parents too much about school anymore. On the day I finished my first year, which was celebrated with a party for all the students and their families, I decided not to tell my parents about it. I seriously could not believe that they would find this important because they didn't accept my choice of course at all. When they found out that I hadn't told them about the party, they were very angry with me and ignored me the whole summer vacation long.

During this time of study, things got harder and harder for me. Yet I did find my way in the student house. I wasn't one of the newbies anymore, so it was MY house! I really liked the people living on my floor. We did a lot of things together, so I felt comfortable with them. My fear of people, however, stayed and got even worse. I felt so unhappy, yet I couldn't explain why. I struggled with my internships in particular. The work wasn't too difficult and I was good at it, but when it was time for evaluation, I would always burst into tears, even though I knew I had done well. I just couldn't cope with those evaluations as it felt like people were going to judge me again. I feared they would tell me that I wasn't good enough.

There was a lot going on in my mind and I didn't know how to make sense of or solve the mental turmoil I was experiencing. I withdrew into a made-up fantasy world and started to tell stories to my mentor in school that were not (entirely) true. I also shared these stories with one of my roommates. I got more and more tangled in my web of lies and had no idea anymore about how I could get out of this. I did realise one thing however: I needed help, but I didn't have a clue about where or how to ask for it, so I continued to struggle and to lie.

At the end of my third school year I told my mentor that I had attempted suicide during the Christmas break (which was not true). She told me that she couldn't help me anymore and that I needed professional help. My heart leapt for joy. Professional help was exactly what I needed, but for entirely different reasons than those known by my mentor.

So, I went to a psychologist who worked together with my school. He told me during the first meeting that he would keep my mentor posted on our conversations. I really liked my mentor and I knew she liked me too. I didn't want to jeopardise this. It was so nice to have someone I really liked, and who really liked me, so I didn't want to lose her. So I did not see another way aside from continuing my lies.

My relationship with my boyfriend was not going very smoothly at this time. I started to get more and more annoyed with him. The way he walked, the way he moved, the way he shuffled his feet, how he laughed, and even the way he breathed. Of course, these were all things that he couldn't do anything about! We argued more and more frequently. I already knew at that point that he was not the one for me, not the person with whom I wanted to grow old with. Yet, I didn't dare to end our relationship, as that would mean that I would lose my safe, huge human teddy bear. So I didn't make any decisions related to this part of my life either.

During the last year of my study, I had to start to think about what it was that I wanted to do next. My options were to start working or to sign up for another course. Furthermore, if I were to choose another course, which one should that be? When I tried to imagine myself working, I immediately started to panic. I had become so insecure about myself that I was convinced I would not be good enough to do any job. But starting another course?? Which one was I going to choose?

All this thinking or, rather, worrying, didn't make me any happier. The sessions I had with the school psychologist weren't making me any happier either, because I felt kind of obliged to keep lying, and I felt more and more guilty every day. I really didn't know what to do! One thing I knew for sure: things needed to change, because if my life continued on the same track, I didn't want to live anymore. But how to change? I didn't have a clue.

I decided to go to Spain to finish my studies. It sounded ideal to me. I decided to go to Barcelona, my favourite city. I was looking forward to being surrounded by the language (which I had been trying to learn after school hours), the beautiful sunny weather, and the lovely environment. So, together with a classmate, I got on the coach to Barcelona.

While there, I felt great. The sun shining on my head made me feel better. But the thinking and worrying didn't stop in Spain. It continued just like it had been at home.

One day, my roommates and I went to Montserat, a monastery in the hills around Barcelona. It was really beautiful there. However, as I have a slight disgust of the Catholic Church and everything associated with it, I decided to go for a walk while my friends visited the church. During my walk I came across some statues (I guess it was the Via Crucis, the Way of the Cross). When I passed a certain statue I stopped at the edge of the path. I was looking into the valley and thinking, "If I jump now, everything will be over and everything will be solved." At that point, a very loud, low-toned man's voice yelled into my ear in Spanish: "Well, why don't you jump?!?".

I was scared to death and immediately turned around to see who was talking to me, but I couldn't see anyone. I looked into the valley again and heard the voice yell for a second time: "What are you waiting for? Come on, jump!". I turned around again, but I still couldn't see anyone, so I started to run as fast as I could towards the monastery, back to the crowds of people. I was really terrified.

This voice stayed with me. He spoke both Spanish and Dutch to me. He told me to do things. For example, he told me to buy ten kilograms of washing powder and said that if I refused to do this, he would harm my little nephew. I really loved my nephew, he meant the world to me, so I would have done everything within my power to prevent him from getting hurt. So I bought those ten kilograms of washing powder, although we didn't even have a washing machine!

This is a pretty innocent example but, quite soon after this, things got less innocent. This voice told me to kill myself. He also told me to hurt my roommate while she was sleeping. I was terrified of this voice and found it really difficult to resist the things he told me to do like killing myself (but apparently I did resist killing myself, otherwise I would not be writing this book now). Instead of killing myself, I started to hurt myself: hitting my fists and banging my head against the wall. Then the voice was quiet for a very short time. But he always came up with something else that I had to do and my nephew was always the ransom ("If you don't do what I say, you will never see him alive again.")

A couple of weeks after this voice started to talk to me, my boyfriend came to Barcelona to visit me. He had to save a lot of money to get there and had decided to visit me for a week. I was thrilled and excited. I was at the airport way too early to pick up him up. I really wanted to see him and thought that meant I was no longer annoyed by all those tiny things about him. I thought we could start over.

But as soon as he arrived and we were on our way back to the city, I immediately started to get annoyed again. The voice got involved in it too. I can't exactly remember what he was saying, but all of his comments were about me and about how I wasn't treating my boyfriend correctly. This voice said things like I wasn't being fair to him, that I was leading him on, and that I didn't deserve him.

The things I was hearing did not make me happy at all, but it never crossed my mind, not for a second, to tell anyone.

During the second night of my boyfriend's stay, things went wrong. The things the voice was saying had such an impact on me and on my thinking. I knew the voice was right, that I wasn't being fair as I already knew that this was not the man I could see myself growing old with. Yet I stayed with him because I did love him and feared the alternative. The voice said that I did not deserve my boyfriend, and I came to the conclusion that he deserved better than me - he deserved something (or someone) better, someone who did want to grow old with him. So, after having another argument that night, I broke up with him. Neither of us saw this coming at all.

My boyfriend didn't have money to change his flight or his accommodation, so he stayed in our apartment, laughing with my roommates but completely ignoring me. I felt completely worthless, but at least the voice shut up about this subject.

I untangled more knots whilst in Spain. I decided that I didn't want to start working yet because I was convinced that I would not be able to manage it. I also came to this choice due to another reason that was more important to me. One of the reasons I started this Social Work course was because I wanted to find out what was wrong with me. My whole life I had felt different to the people around me, but I didn't know what it was that made me different. I still hadn't found the answer to that question, but I was still wondering about it. So I hoped to find the answer in my next course: psychology.

When that knot was untangled, I wrote a letter to the school psychologist to tell him that I would finish my studies soon and would no longer be able to pay him. I asked for a referral to the Riagg (ambulatory mental health services). I hoped that with this referral I could finally start with a clean slate and would be able to tell the truth about my problems (talking about the voice I was hearing didn't even cross my mind).

So, I returned to the Netherlands with my final paper, written in three languages and with five voices in my head (during my time in Spain, three other voices appeared, but as they are no longer present I won't go into detail about them here).

On the day I got my diploma, I also had my first intake meeting with a psychologist. I felt quite ambivalent about this. I had the letter of referral from the school psychologist which was full of the lies I had told him. I didn't know what to do: continue the story of lies, but then it didn't make sense to go to this meeting; or go there and confess that things were a bit different than the way they were written about in that letter.

After weighing up all of the pros and cons and enduring the many, "Liar, liar, pants on fire" remarks from the voice, I decided to write a letter explaining what the real situation was. I wanted to read this letter out loud during the intake meeting. This decision prompted a, "That's the spirit!" remark from the voice.

I told the psychologist that I needed help with my lying. I didn't tell him about the voices, even when he directly asked me about it. I also didn't speak about it as I found the question rather strange: "Do you hear voices that aren't there?". I thought that was a silly question, because if I was hearing something, then it would be there, otherwise I would not be hearing it. So I answered in the negative to this question.

In the meantime, a new life had started for me. I had moved to a new student home with a total of four people, two of whom were hardly there. I began a new course at the university, which was only six hours of lessons a week (at most). The rest of the time I was free to study on my own. This was very hard for me. I had way too much time to think and to worry. Although I hated my old student home at the beginning, now there was no one at home I could talk to or laugh with. My head started to overflow with worries and the voices got worse. They were there all the time, threatening me, telling me to do stuff and it was no longer innocent!

Everything they said came down to the fact that I had to kill myself, because that would be better for me and for the rest of the world. I constantly told them to piss off, to leave me alone, and to go and mess with someone else. But the louder I told them, the more they (and especially this voice) told me to do stuff. They told me that I had to jump off a bridge, that I had to walk on the train tracks, that I had to walk on the motorway. And every time they added a threat with it: if I did not do as I was told, they would harm (or even kill) my nephew. Although I am not stupid, these threats made me search for ways to kind of do what they told me to do. I was looking for compromises and started searching for alternatives. I didn't kill myself, but instead I hurt myself. Then the voice was silent for a moment. But the assignments came more regularly, and the times of hurting myself got more frequent and more serious.

It felt like I was slowly giving up control over my life. It felt as though I didn't have a life of my own anymore. The voices determined my life and, shortly after this, they became my life. Me and my own will no longer existed. It felt as though myself and my life were entirely in the voices' hands.

This led, one evening, to a taxi driver dragging me off a bridge, as I was sitting there waiting for my chance to jump on the motorway and die. I ended up being admitted to the Crisis Centre in the city centre of my home town.

Even while I was in the Crisis Centre, the voices didn't leave me alone. Yet I still didn't tell anyone that I was hearing voices. During my new course I was taught by the textbooks that hearing voices was a symptom of schizophrenia and that the treatment of schizophrenia was mainly comprised of medication, being admitted to psychiatric wards, and the quality of life getting worse and worse. So I kept my mouth shut about it. That was not going to happen to me!

I became so out of control and unpredictable with the staff that they could no longer guarantee the other patients' safety or my own. So they called my crisis manager (a psychiatrist), who came over to the centre to talk to me after his working hours. This psychiatrist had been my crisis manager for quite a while and I knew that I could talk to him as a human being. I also knew that he was specialised in hearing voices, as he had given a lecture on the subject during my studies.

I can't exactly remember how it happened, but I guess at one point he asked me whether I was hearing voices or not. And without thinking about the consequences I said: "Yes". I do remember very well my conviction that my answer would mean the end of the world, or at least the end of MY world. I would be locked up in the psychiatric hospital, I would be stuffed with medication, I would probably have to say goodbye to my new room and my new course etc.

But that didn't happen. Instead, he responded in a really quiet and 'normal' manner. He asked me how many voices I was hearing. He also asked whether they were men or women and if I knew them. I did think at that point that it was quite odd, but because he reacted in a normal way and didn't freak out about it, I calmed down and dared to say something about the voices, even though they told me not to do so. They were afraid this man was going to try everything to get rid of them, and that didn't seem like a good idea to them.

Then something happened that drastically changed my worldview: the crisis manager asked me if he could talk to my voices. I remember thinking: "Which one of us is crazy now???" The voice inside my head answered. The crisis manager understood that something was going on and he asked me what was happening. I told him that the voice had said "Yes" and he asked me if I would agree to this conversation between him and the voice. To be honest, I had no idea of what to think of it at that point but I agreed.

One of the first questions he asked was if the voice had a name. The voice's answer was: "It's not important who I am, it is important that I'm here." But he did agree to me giving him a name.

This conversation made it clear that the voice was there to help me. He had already been with me for a very long time and he noticed that I had great difficulties with making decisions and that I was suffering because of this. He wanted to help me. He wanted me to make a choice and to act upon the choice I made. He was mainly referring to my fear of living and believed that I had to make a decision about this. It didn't matter to him what my choice would be -dying or living - but if I were to choose death then I should definitely end my life. If I chose to live, then I had to go for life, to start living fully and to stop these halfway attempts to end my life.

The voice also explained to the crisis manager that he was using 'reverse psychology' on me. As he had been with me for a very long time, he knew that I was as stubborn as hell and that no one could tell me what to do. If someone would tell me to go left, I would go right. So his 'style' was based on this fact: by saying to me that I should kill myself, he hoped that it would made me choose life. The crisis manager asked him if he thought I understood his tactics. He came to the conclusion that I did not. So there was work to do. We had to find a mutual language that we could both understand.

The name I gave this voice was 'De Brutaalste', which means something like 'The Most Rude One' as he was the one who was always answering first and took leadership in a kind of brutal way. You could also say that he's 'The Cheeky One'. He didn't disagree on that name, it seemed more like he felt kind of proud of it.
I wasn't sent off to the psychiatric hospital that night, but I was sent home with an appointment with the crisis manager (in his role as my psychiatrist) in his office the very next day.

During the months that followed, the psychiatrist explained to me how I could talk to my voices. We started to look further into when the voices came, why they came, what they were like (their characteristics) and what or who they might represent. We used the Maastricht Interview* to do so. That was not so easy for me as it meant that I had to start to really listen to the voices, not being scared, and not taking the first response as the one and only truth. I had to learn how to ask deeper questions, to show respect, and demand respect in return. I also had to start looking at my life and what had happened. This was something I hadn't dared to do up until this point.

It was also really important for me to take back control over my life. If I could somehow 'control' the voices (meaning that I would create a different relationship with them), it would naturally follow that I would get more control over my life again.

To make a very long story a bit short(er)...
For a very long time I saw 'De Brutaalste' as my worst enemy. He could literally make or break me. He knew what my weakest points were and would poke at these whenever he could. When he did, I ended up in my, "I'm worthless, I can't do anything, I'm no use" mode.
But because I began to learn how to really listen to him, and also how to set my boundaries, the relationship with him changed over time. I stopped seeing him as my worst enemy and instead as a good advisor that I could ask for help when I was faced with a dilemma.
The way 'De Brutaalste' was speaking changed during the day. He started to speak in stand-up comedy and movie quotes more and more often, two things that I really loved (stand up comedy and movies). He was changing how he spoke to me from morning to evening.
His remarks during the daytime were usually very cryptic. I really liked this as I had to think hard about what he meant. But during our daily 'consulting hour' (in the evening - when the voices had an opportunity to discuss things that were really important to them), where I really had to listen and to try to understand him, he spoke in normal, day-to-day sentences.

Today I can say that 'De Brutaalste' is one of my best friends. This has made me doubt whether I should change his name. He has also

told me that his name no longer applies to him and had come from a time when I had negative associations of him.
I have told him that these negative associations have been gone for years and that, to me, this is just his name now, nothing more, nothing less. I have also told him that changing his name now would not feel ok to me. He helped me while listening to this name and I am really grateful and proud of that. At the same time, I don't want to forget how things were very different, less natural, once. To me his name is an honour to what was and what is.

If you were to ask me what I think 'De Brutaalste's' function/role is, I would say that he helps me to make choices and to stay committed to the choices I have made. He's a helper and a protector. Besides that, he's just a friend I can have a good time with, who I can chat to and have a laugh with, who is always there and who I don't want to lose.

He came for the first time when I was in Spain, and when I returned to Spain years later, in 2009, he specifically asked me to go to the exact spot where he spoke for the very first time. He asked me to bring matches, pen and paper. So I did.

I will finish this chapter about 'De Brutaalste' with the literal text (the reason for the pen and paper) of the conversation I (I) had with him (B) at that spot.

Sunday, September 6, 2009

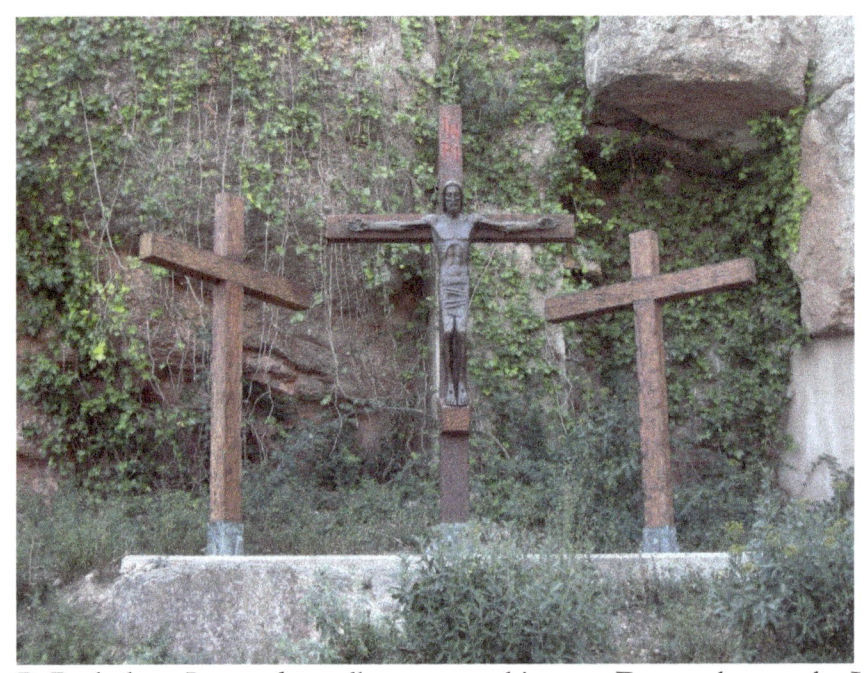

B: Back then, I started to talk to you at this spot. Do you know why I picked this spot?

I: No, I guess because you could challenge me there?

B: That too, but that's not the only reason. What is it that you see in front of you?

I: A part of the Via Crucis.

B: Sure, but which part?

I: The crucifixion of Jesus?

B: Well done, you paid attention back then. At least those cosy religious lessons brought some fruits. Back to my story. The crucifixion of Jesus. You know, I had been watching you and had been with you for a very long time before I started to speak to you. I was already there when you went to pre-school. In pre-school you were a scared little birdie. You were sitting under the table and hardly came out of your hiding spot. The teachers thought you were extremely shy, but you were afraid. Afraid and exhausted as you hardly slept as you had to stay alert all the time… and you had every reason to do so. I watched over you, but I didn't do anything, except that I used one of your talents: your fantasy. You developed or created invisible friends and I helped these friends to help you. You do remember these friends, don't you?

I: Of course.

B: Ok, back to the point where I took over. You sent your friends away and the result was that you were incredibly lonely during High School. Even if you would have liked to share things with someone, you didn't have anyone to share it with. That's why you started to beg for attention in every possible (sometimes really weird) way.

I: That's right, but High School is way before your arrival…

B: Polle Polle (Swahili, meaning something like, 'Slow down')! I will get to that point soon. Up until then your life was a bit similar to the Via Crucis. You both literally and figuratively suffered from the 'heavy cross' that your home situation had put on your shoulders. You always walked around with your head bent towards the floor, staring at the floor.

During your Social Work studies, within this huge group of people, you felt even lonelier and unhappier. You were so unhappy that you had no idea anymore of what you wanted. You doubted yourself. You found yourself so despicable that you thought you did not deserve to live. You didn't think you had the right to live. And that was totally unfair.

You are not the one who is bad, you are not despicable, disgusting or anything else that you think you are. You think you are too evil to be loved or, even worse, that you are not capable of loving anyone, but that's bullshit. Wake up baby! You ARE love, that's the reason you survived. The voices didn't do that, you did!

I: No I didn't…

B: Shut up and listen! You are not evil. You are capable of immensely enjoying things and loving people. That's what makes you different from your Mum. You love other people, sincerely and without a doubt, everyone except yourself. Your Mum just loves herself and the rest is not important. The inability to love yourself is literally and figuratively destroying you.
While you were here in Spain, your desperation was higher than it ever was before. I had to do something, I had to intervene and exactly at this spot at that moment. Either you would die here at the cross or you would rise like a Phoenix from the ashes and start living. I dared you: jump off the cliff and die or turn around and live.
    I: Well, it was not exactly a choice: you only gave me one option.
B: Yes and just like I expected you to, you chose the option I didn't mention, but I admit, that was a dangerous experiment for me to try. You chose life, but made things even worse for yourself. You chased away the one person you really loved. You pushed him aside and withdrew even more. You became totally convinced to never trust anyone ever again.
But you also asked for help, so you did make a choice. Finally, you did something and you really tried, even though you still doubted yourself on that. I'm proud of you, but you need to start being proud of yourself.
    I: But I'm not...
B: Time to change! You can change that. Turn this little flame that's already there into a huge bonfire.
    I: I wish I knew how to do so.
B: You don't need to know yet, time will tell!!

B: Something else. I was gone for a while and I think I owe you an explanation. I wanted to see if you could make it on your own. With all the upcoming changes, when saying goodbye and starting over, all alone, were major themes, I wanted to see how you would react.
    I: Well, I screwed that one up pretty well!

B: No you didn't, I was the one who made a mistake, wrong again babe! I picked the wrong moment, a moment where everything came at you at once and if everything comes at once, you can't handle it. That has always been the case and it probably will stay that way.

I: So you are saying that I did well?

B: Well, let's put it like this: it was very clear that you couldn't handle the situation, but that's ok. You are not ready for my departure yet. For now, there's enough on your plate.

I: Do you have to go, in the end?

B: I don't have to do anything, just like you. If you want me to go, I will go. If you want me to stay, I will stay. I just wanted to see if you would make it on your own.

*I: Are you also 'The Polar Bear'**?*

B: No, that's someone you do and don't know, but that's something you have to clear with him. Don't be too scared.

I: Sometimes I don't want to know.

B: And sometimes you do, so just ask! The Via Crucis -you came off the cross that day and you tried to rise from the ashes like the Phoenix, but you are not showing any progress on that anymore, on the contrary. If you were Felix the Phoenix*** I would say you have some trouble getting out of that pile of ash. And that's what I want you to do, you have to solve some issues, so you can move on.

I: Like?

B: I want you to stop feeling guilty towards your parents. You made mistakes, they made mistakes. The difference is that you were a kid and they were the adults. But in many ways you were the wise one. I want you to be the wisest again. I want you to join them on their trip abroad.

I: Why?

B: Because you would not be able to live with yourself if something happened to them and you hadn't been trying to talk to them. Try to use the time that is left with them as well as possible and I want to help you with that.

I: What exactly do you mean?

B: "I am I and you are you and that's how they do things". I want you to open up more to people. Give them the benefit of the doubt. Try to trust people.
I: I really do try to do that now as well!
B: Then try a little harder. It will never be the same as when you were a kid. You are an adult now, you can perfectly well stand up for yourself and be assertive if needed. People love you, care about you, and trust you, even when they know your background. Don't you think it would only be fair to give them a chance?
I: But I find it so incredibly difficult to believe that people mean it, to believe that they really care about me.
B: That's because you don't believe it yourself. You have been brainwashed, but you are allowed to believe in yourself now.
I: Yes, but that's fucking difficult!
B: It sure is, I won't deny that, but you can ask the people around you to help you.
I: But how?
B: Do you remember that someone gave you a 'positive things' booklet once? Well, make a 'positive you' book!
I: And what would that look like? I would be finished within 10 seconds.
B: And that's why you should ask other people to help you. Ask them to write down, on a piece of paper, what it is that they like about you or why they appreciate you. Put the pieces of paper in a folder and every time you feel bad or worthless about yourself, you can re-read them.
I: It's stupid to ask for that...
B: Yeah sure, incredibly stupid. Feeling bad about yourself is way better!
I: No, you are right, but how do I ask people to do this? I'm not 5 years old where I could ask people, smiling my best smile, to write in my friend's book.
B: Use me perhaps? Just tell them I have given you an assignment.

I: lol... You do know that I have been taught not to do the things you tell me to do...
B: Yeah sure! And you always follow the rules and do as you are told. Just do it. You will see that some people even like doing it, but there might be some people that will say no to it, that's possible.
I: Ok. Why did you ask me to bring the matches?
B: I wanted to let you 'burn your past' so you could rise from the ashes, but it's too dry up here. We don't want to burn down Montserat, do we?
I: Well, lol, it is still a Catholic institution...
B: Yes that's true... Tempting but no thanks.
I: I'm glad you are back.
B: It's good to have a real conversation with you again. We do not do that often enough, but Lesley**** needs some more time right now. To lose Mum and Dad for the second time is very difficult for her. You need to guide her in this process. If you guide her, you might be able to become a bit more independent yourself.
I: I don't understand what you mean by that.
B: That's alright, you might understand it some day. Have faith in yourself and in others, that's my message for now. You are doing a great job!
I: Ok, can I please go down now, I'm freezing!
B: You sissy!

* to put it simply, the Maastricht Interview for voice hearers is a structured interview which is used to get to know the voices better. It was developed by Professor Marius Romme and Dr Sandra Escher.
** another voice
*** the Phoenix from the Harry Potter stories, my favourite books, written by J.K. Rowling
**** another voice

De Jankende Hond
('The Howling Dog')

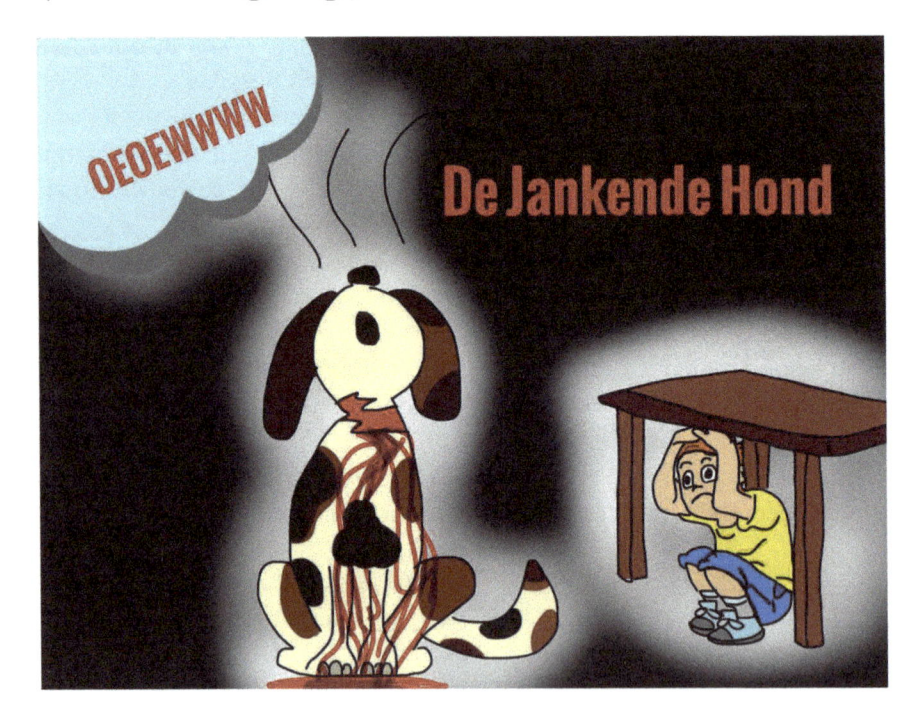

This chapter is not suitable for people with a weak stomach. But it is an important chapter to include in order to understand the disturbed environment I was growing up in. It also explains why I needed my invisible friends and my fantasy world so badly to survive. But a warning is definitely in order.

When I was five years old, we moved to a new house. This meant that I was living further from my school and also from the few friends I had. We didn't exactly live in a fancy neighbourhood and this, combined with the fact that it was further from school, meant that my friends never came to visit. My brother and I had to play together as there were not a lot of kids in our part of the neighbourhood.

Things were not very nice at home. My Mum was really unpredictable, so home didn't feel like a safe place to me. Since I could never predict what was right and what was wrong (because this was changing every minute), I got punished a lot. Punishment could mean all kind of things but, to summarise it, you could say it was abuse. Some people have even called it torture, but I still find that very hard to say.

In our old house my punishment usually meant me being locked up in a cupboard under the stairs. I found that horrible because as soon as the doors closed it was dark and I could not see anything. But I could hear all kind of noises I couldn't make any sense of and I felt all kind of things crawling on me. It wasn't so much the dark that I was afraid of, it was the spiders, and the darkness meant I could not see the spiders.

By moving to the new house, the locking up in the cupboard came to an end, simply because the new house did not have such a cupboard. However, unfortunately for me, the new house contained an even better spot for punishment: the shed.
Though, to me, the shed was less scary than the cupboard. At least it wasn't that dark and I had more space to move around. There were all kind of tools that I could play with and the best thing was that our dog lived in the shed as well!

We had a large breed of dog. And when I say large, I really mean large: the dog was taller than me! My dog was my best buddy. I told him all of my worries and secrets and he pretended to understand me. In fact our dog was deaf, so he couldn't even hear what I was saying, but I was convinced that he heard me and understood everything I had to say.
My dog slept on a wooden plateau in the shed. He also had his food and water in there. When I was being locked up for longer periods of

time, the dog didn't have a problem with sharing his food, drink and bed with me.
The dog was my best friend, together with the invisible friends (voices) inside my head that helped me through these difficult times by playing language-related games with me, making jokes and giving me useful tips.

When I was six years old, my Dad told my Mum that he was going to leave her and that he would take us kids with him. My Mum didn't like that idea very much, so she glared at him and said: "Look what will happen if you do so". By the way, I didn't know about this until a couple of years ago, but this does 'explain' the event that followed on from this.

The day after my Dad's announcement, he had to work as usual and that meant he would return home around dinner time. I went to school during the day but, as soon as I returned home, I ended up in the shed again.
About an hour before my Dad was due to come home, my Mum violently dragged me out of the shed and into the house. I could see in her eyes that something bad was about to happen, but you could never really predict what she might do. She was muttering to herself with this vague, threatening look in her eyes.

My brother and I were pushed into the house and were told to stay in the living room. We were hiding under the table together, both terrified, while my Mum fetched the dog. The dog didn't exactly cooperate. It was as though he could sense what was about to happen, but my Mum hit and kicked him into the house.

Once we all were inside, she grabbed a huge cooking knife and a plastic bowl. The dog was lying down in front of the table, between my brother and I on one side and my Mum on the other side. A growl regularly came from his throat. My Mum didn't seem to hear this. She grabbed the dog's head really tightly and, as he started to howl, she muttered: "This will teach him."

The next moment, she slit my dog's throat and collected the blood in the bowl. I remember that neither my brother nor I were able to make a sound. My brother wet himself and I did what I always (automatically) did when my Mum was in a mood like this: I was no longer in my body, but was floating above it, looking down from a distance at what my Mum was doing.

As the bleeding stopped, she grabbed me from under the table and pushed the bowl powerfully to my mouth. I was terrified and didn't understand what it was that she wanted. She told us that we had to drink the blood of this innocent, slaughtered animal, so we "would stay innocent forever". I tried to resist with all the power in me, but she pinched my nose so in order to inhale I needed to open my mouth to be able to breathe. That's how a gulp of warm blood entered my mouth and that was so horrible that I immediately puked my guts out. Until today I can't stand the taste and the smell of blood, it makes me feel sick.

My brother responded almost in the same way as me. He also puked his guts out.
Perhaps it is unnecessary to tell you that the dog didn't survive this.
When my Dad returned home, it was already dark. He hardly spoke. He grabbed the dog off the floor and disappeared. He left and only returned a few days later, without the dog. For all of this time he left us alone with my Mum, whose usual vague, scary look in her eyes was even scarier and more threatening than usual - combined with the huge smile that was painted on her face.

The howling sound my dog made, just before his throat was slit, has always stayed with me. In moments when I'm exhausted, or terrified, I will start to hear this sound again. It will also happen when I have the gut feeling that something bad is going to happen, when I sense danger or when I feel very unsafe.

It took me quite a while before I could explain this sound. The connection with the last sound I ever heard from my dog was not too difficult (but telling someone else about it was a different thing), but finding out what it meant was not so easy for me.

I'm not very good with emotions. Emotions were something that only my Mum was allowed to have in our house. No one else was allowed to feel anything.
As soon as we showed the slightest sign of an emotion other than 'neutral' we would be punished. In this way, I unlearned the showing of emotions. After a while, I didn't even have a clue what it was that I felt in my body.

It took me years before I finally understood that it was fear and the feeling of not being safe that caused me to hear this sound.

The sound still works like some kind of signal: as soon as I start to hear it (I call it a voice), I have to soul-search and think really hard. Apparently, something is going on. What is it that frightens me? Why do I feel unsafe?
As soon as I start to think about it and to look deeper into it, it usually doesn't take very long before I know what it is that is causing my distress.

I don't think it needs any explanation why I, and therefore also the youngest voices, are obsessed with dogs and why I/we can't cope when someone is not treating a dog with respect.

Lesley

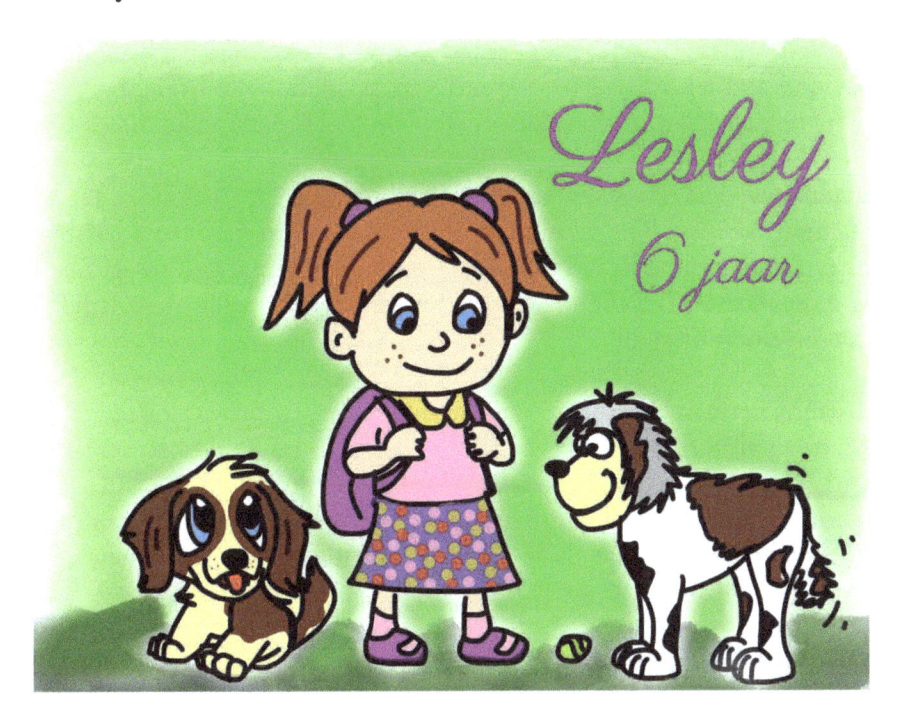

As a kid I went through a lot. I was abused and neglected from a very young age and I learnt, really young, that I was not allowed to show my emotions. As emotions were not permitted, I never learned the words attached to these emotions. Talking about the way I felt was not an option. I also didn't learn how to cope with these feelings and emotions in a normal, healthy way.

There was no time or space to be afraid or sad. I just had to go on and to make sure that I would survive. That was easiest by not feeling anything and just getting on with things. I had to adjust to everything and everyone and to try to be as invisible as possible.

I also learnt from a young age to be hyper-alert. As soon as I entered a room, I could figure out instantly what was going on, who could be trusted, and who could not. I could instantly sense who was safe to be around and who I had to stay as far as possible away from. This is a very useful skill to have while growing up in a situation like mine.

I was raised as a boy, except for the times when my extended family came to visit us. The whole time I was told not to act like a girl but, when family came to visit, I was dressed as a girl and had to act like a girl, even though I didn't have a clue about how to do that! I didn't understand this at all!

I cannot remember, outside of these times when my extended family came to visit, that I have ever felt the desire to be a girl or to act like a girl. Yet, when I try to understand Lesley and to look at the things she likes and loves, I do think that I somehow might have had the desire to be a bit girly. That there might be a little girl in me somewhere, deep down inside.

As a young kid I loved our dog. He was my best friend. It would have been difficult not to be friends as we spent a lot of time together. Our dog slept in the shed and I spent a lot of my time in that same shed (not on a voluntary basis by the way). While I was locked up in the shed, I did not always get food or drink, but the dog didn't mind sharing its food and water with me. During that period, the dog and my Granny were my best buddies. These were the two creatures I trusted unconditionally.

When I was six years old, the dog got killed in a horrible way in front of my eyes, as I told you about in the last chapter. That's an image (or, to put it a bit better, a little movie) that will never leave my memory. Even as an adult, it still affects me.

As a kid I loved stories. I still do. I could write and read from a very early age, from the age of three to be precise. I read books at a pace faster than lightning. I read mainly fairy tales and magical stories, but also stories about cool boys, animals and (also) happy, lovely girls with loving parents.

I can't remember exactly when it started, but one day I heard a crying child. That's not uncommon as the world is full of (crying) children. You can find them anywhere: on the streets, in the house above, next to, behind or on another floor of your apartment. Everywhere!
But when this sound continued day and night and followed me everywhere I went, it started to get annoying and I became frustrated. It took me a while to realise that this sound had developed inside my head and not so much from the outside world.

During this period I 'lost time' on a regular basis. What I mean is that there were huge gaps in my memory. I had no idea what had happened or what I had done. Those periods were pretty frightening, but I just laughed it off when people asked me about it, pretending that it was nothing and was the most normal thing in the world. I also didn't really want to think about what was happening, or to have a closer look at these time gaps, as I feared that knowing might be worse than not knowing.

It also happened regularly that I 'woke up' in a place and had no idea where I was or how I got there. These moments scared me to death. Something was happening I could not explain. Such things that I don't understand or can't explain make me anxious and angry. Even though I didn't know in those moments where I was and what I was doing in that place, I persistently refused to ask people for help. I didn't ask people where I was, how long I had been there and what I was doing there. I took all the uncertainty for granted and ploughed all of my efforts into getting back home. I tried to forget about these events as quickly as possible. During moments like this, the sound of crying in my head was very loud and very persistent.

One day I 'woke up' in my own house. On the floor there was a plastic bag with girls clothing in a very tiny size, in horrible shades of pink and with lots of sparkles on them. There also was a colouring book opened at a picture of a dog, coloured in (or, rather, scratched on) with blue marker.
My left hand was covered in blue stains. The same colour as the dog in the colouring book.
I didn't understand what was happening and I became very scared. This couldn't have anything to do with me, could it? I was right-handed and I hated the colour pink, let alone sparkles!
I tore the picture up and threw it in the bin (the crying started again) and I began to wash my hands to get rid of the blue stains. I returned the clothing (more and louder crying) and again I tried really hard to forget about this incident. But I didn't manage to forget it.

I knew what a 'multiple personality' was but, at the same time, I didn't believe in this. I didn't believe that there could be more than one part within one person and that someone could change into someone else and do things they couldn't remember. I had seen something about it on television once, but to me it looked and felt so fake. Yet I could no longer deny that there was something strange going on with me and that strange things were happening I couldn't remember.

It was during this time that I discovered (with a little help) that this crying kid had a name: her name was Lesley and she was a 'big girl' (according to herself) and was six years old. She did sound much younger though, but was very insistent on being six years old.

From the moment I knew her name, I was told to be kind to her, to take care of her and to comfort her when she was crying or when something changed in her behaviour. The crying began to decrease and she started to talk more and more.

Lesley loves dogs and she gets totally upset when a dog is looking sad (and believe me, dogs have a special talent for looking sad). When a dog is looking sad, that is (in her eyes) due to the fact that someone is hurting the dog or is not being kind to the dog.
If it was up to her, she would pet every dog that we meet in the streets. While walking in the streets she greets every dog, and I mean EVERY dog, with a, "hello dog". This might sound really cute, but when you start counting the amount of dogs you will pass from home to work for example, you might get an idea of how many times this ritual repeats itself (and believe me when I say that Lesley can spot dogs from a mile away).

Other animals can't be hurt either, not even the animals she's really scared of (like spiders, cats, horses, flies, mosquitoes, bees, wasps, actually everything that isn't a dog or a bear). And this is also the case for all the stuffed toy animals we have in the house, but most of all her own two toy animals. If one of her toy dogs falls out of the bed during the night, she will start to cry hysterically and is convinced that my stuffed Hippo pushed her dog out of the bed and is "not very kind!".

Lesley will take things she hears very literally. Once she had a conversation with my psychiatrist (I wasn't there, she took over) during which he used a word that was too difficult for her. It won't make any sense to translate this into English but I will try to describe the consequences of such a situation.
Lesley started to ask me questions about what she had heard, but I could not answer and she got frustrated. She kept repeating the same question over and over again for weeks and I couldn't answer her. I asked the psychiatrist, but he didn't have a clue about what Lesley was talking about. So she got even more frustrated. As I had no idea of

how to solve this situation, I got frustrated too. I became so frustrated that I started to bang my head against the wall, hoping this would make her, her stupid questions, and her hysterical crying go away. But of course it didn't work that way.

Weeks later I listened to the tape of that psychiatry session (as I tended to dissociate a lot and lose time during our conversations, we started to tape the sessions). After listening to the tape, I finally understood what Lesley was asking about. It was a difficult word that she had divided into the sounds. Now her question did make sense and as I told the psychiatrist we started to laugh. Now I can laugh about situations like that, but at that point in time I found it really complicated.

Lesley also has some very persistent language 'mistakes'. For example, she will always say 'daughter' when she means 'doctor'. The other examples are difficult to translate as they won't make sense in English. But to give you some English equivalents of the kind of things Lesley takes very literally: if someone said that it is raining cats and dogs outside, Lesley would run to the window and start looking hopefully for cats and dogs falling from the sky. Or if someone says, "That's a hard nut to crack" she will go to look for the nut!

Rik and Roy* really like how naive Lesley still is. They love to play on her naivety and to pull pranks on her. For example, they told her that there is a dog living in the iPad called 'Ok'. To make sure that she would believe their story, they changed the wallpaper on my iPad to a Beagle dog. 'Ok' will start to bark every once in a while and they have told Lesley that when he starts to bark, he's feeling sad and lonely and wants to be petted on the nose really gently. They told her that if she would do so, 'Ok' would stop barking.

To clarify (in case you don't understand yet!), the sound of my alarm clock on the iPad is a barking dog sound. So, as soon as the alarm goes off and 'Ok' starts barking, Lesley starts frantically saying: "Don't be sad 'Ok', just wait, I'm coming, don't be sad, don't bark."

Everything will be thrown out of my hands, literally, and she will run to the iPad and will pet 'Ok' gently on the nose. Meanwhile the teenagers can (still) hardly stop laughing.

You might wonder why the dog is named 'Ok'? As soon as the alarm starts, there will be a grey pop-up screen over the dog's nose which says, 'Cancel alarm? Press Ok'.

For a while, Roy tried to teach Lesley how to read and write, but in the end he lost his patience with her and ceased his attempts. He sometimes still takes care of her when I lose my patience with her, but he has passed this task more and more to another voice over time: 'The Polar Bear'. Lesley sees 'The Polar Bear' a bit like her Daddy and 'De Lieve Vrouwenstem' as her Mummy.

Another thing I know about Lesley is that she is is almost as tall as an adult Saint Bernard dog.

Lesley is always present, 24/7. This means that it is very necessary for me to set some boundaries with her. If I don't, she drives me insane! She keeps asking 'Why?' questions all the time and she can't cope with the fact that I don't know all the answers to her questions.

Lesley has her own 'consulting hour'. With the older voices, this is one hour a day when I HAVE to listen to them and when I can negotiate things with them. Lesley was always the underdog in these conversations and that made her very sad and angry, as she wanted to talk too. When she didn't get any attention, she would take over (this was the case in the 'colouring book affair'). When this happens, I'm no longer there and she is the one in charge and the one who decides what happens and what doesn't happen.

It took a while, but now we have some rules about being 'the temporary boss'. For example, Lesley can't go out on her own, and she is not allowed to open the door or to pick up the phone. And at those times when I'm already outside when she's taking over, she's not allowed to buy any food without 'The Polar Bear' telling her it's ok to buy it (as I have a severe food allergy). These rules seem to work most of the time.

As I have already mentioned, Lesley has her own 'consulting hour'. This is actually half an hour a day where we do the stuff that she likes. We watch children's television series, listen to children's songs, read fairy tales etc.
For a while there was a famous Dutch television program called 'Fabeltjeskrant'. It's a puppet show with an owl reading the newspaper and telling the animals what is happening in their forest. This was very nice as every part only lasted for five minutes and, at the end, the owl always announced that it was time to close your mouth and eyes and go to sleep.
So my idea was that this would be the end of Lesley's 'consulting hour' and after that she needed to go to sleep (meaning, no talking anymore) and for a while this really worked! But then this programme was cancelled and even Lesley noticed that the television was playing the same story over and over again...

Sometimes Lesley doesn't want to be six years old anymore and she will tell everyone that she is seven today. If I ask her why she is seven today, she usually says: "Being six is boring!" But the next day (or an hour or even a minute later) she's six again. This 'aging' usually appears when Rik is bullying her.

If you were to ask me what Lesley's role is, I think I would say that she is the little Mick. The little Mick who was never allowed to be a kid. The little Mick who was never allowed to be scared or sad, and who was never allowed to be a girl or to act girly.
Lesley is also the part of me that still needs to learn about emotions and to understand that it's ok to have emotions. At the same time, she

is full of emotions and shows them, however inappropriate it might be at the time.

If Lesley is scared or sad, this is a sign for me that I have to do some soul searching to find out what it is, in that moment, that is making me feel scared or sad.

Nowadays Lesley is happier and keeps talking and talking. But when she is scared, sad or angry, she can really drive me insane. I'm still not always able to think as she's thinking and to see the world through her eyes, and I don't always have the patience to find out what is bothering her.

Therefore, you could also say that Lesley is my teacher. She teaches me patience and keeps testing and training my empathic ability.

Even though Lesley drives me crazy from time to time, I would not want to be without her. That would be boring! And there would be so many things I would miss out on, as Lesley sees things that we, as grown ups, can't see anymore!

*two other voices

Conijntje

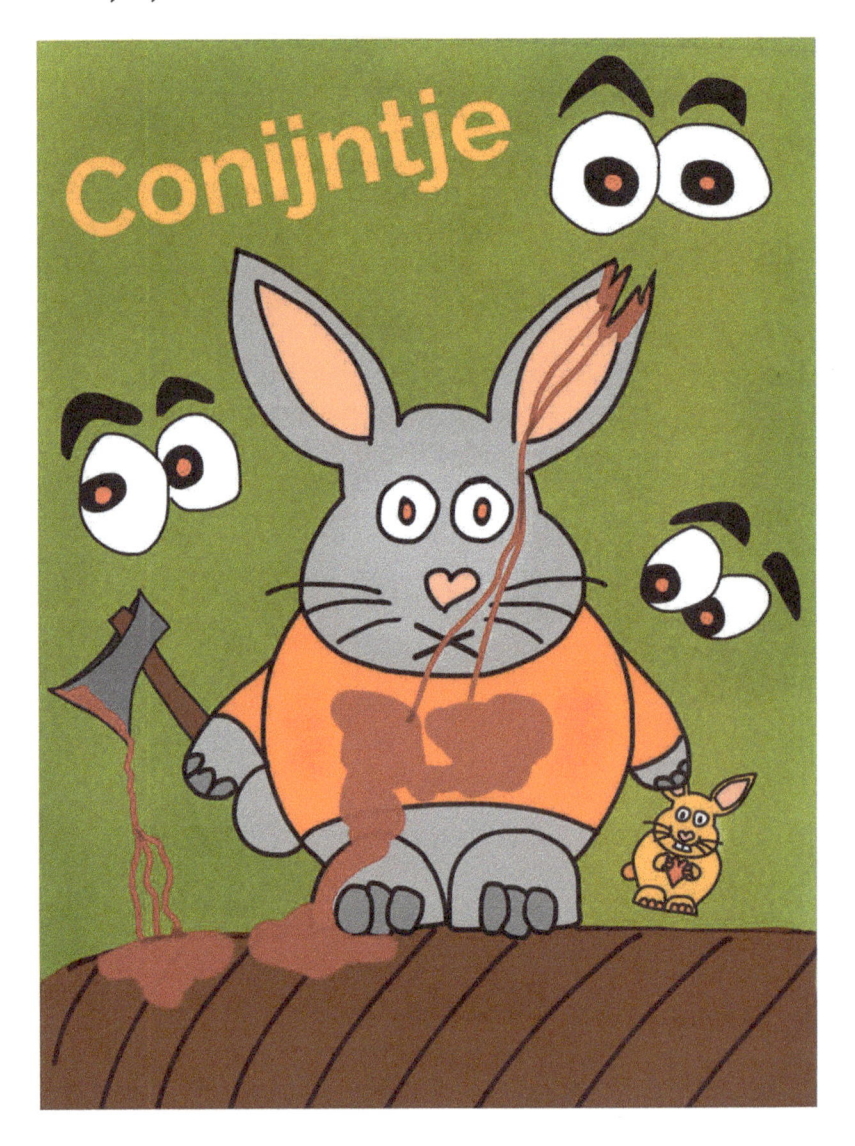

This is a difficult chapter for me to write in more ways than one. And, as if it wasn't difficult enough in Dutch, it's even harder in English. One of these difficulties has something to do with Copyright. I hope that the reader, by using their imagination, will understand what it's actually about without me breaching any Copyright rules. The English equivalent of Conijntje, would be CoMiffy, which right now probably won't make much sense to you as a reader.

If you haven't heard of Miffy, I suggest you might like to Google the name to give you a better understanding of this chapter.

When I was sixteen years old, I was admitted to a child and adolescent psychiatric clinic where I was, up until that moment, an outpatient.

I ended up (as an outpatient) in the clinic as I was continuing to tell lies, and was not supposed to be doing so. As I mentioned before, I had created my own fantasy world. This was necessary for my survival. Today, I think it also has something to do with the fact that, during the few attempts when I tried to tell people about what was going on at home, I always got the same answer: I was told that "Bad things like that could not take place at my home as we were a decent family and my parents were sweet, decent, good people." I was told that I "should not be so silly" and "mustn't talk rubbish about my parents."

So I created (unintentionally, I might add) a 'reality' in which I showed the world my home situation in an adjusted form. I told stories to the people around me I liked and yearned to get attention from (often teachers). After a while, these teachers started to talk to each other about me. They came to the conclusion that the stories I told each of them were not entirely the same. So they called my parents in for a meeting to discuss my behaviour. The consequence was (as this was not the first time) that I was referred to the child and adolescent psychiatric unit. It was decided that I 'was no longer able to distinguish fantasy from reality.

I had to go there on account of my lying. Ironically, however, every time we, as a family, went there I was told: "You will not say anything about what happens here. If you do so, you know where you will sleep tonight." I knew I would end up in the shed again. So I went to these sessions with the message of my Mum in one ear ("don't tell anyone anything") and the questions of the therapists ("please tell us, what is all of this like for you?") in the other ear.

I wanted to please both. I didn't want to betray my parents so I didn't answer the therapists (and felt really guilty about this) and the result was that my Mother got angry with me in front of the therapists saying: "Don't be so rude, answer the questions when you're asked!"
The situation was so unclear and contradicting that I didn't understand what was expected of me. I could never get it right: conforming to the wish of one would be nonconforming to the wish of the other and I felt torn inside. So I (unintentionally) stopped talking altogether. I didn't speak at home, nor in school, nor in the clinic. I kept silent for almost a year!

After almost a year of being silent, I started to talk again during a family therapy session. I shouted at my parents: "I'd rather die than go back home with you." And that felt like the perfect moment to get up and head for the exit. Unfortunately, I ran in the wrong direction towards a dead end and before I reached the end I was pinned down by six adults.

While five of these adults were sitting on top of me trying to calm me down, one of them went to talk to my therapists as it was clear by my spectacular breaking-of-the-silence that something needed to happen. My Dad was asked to try to control me and calm me down. While he was sitting on top of me, pinning me down (I was heavily resisting), for the first time in my life I saw him crying.

I felt horrible and really guilty that I was doing this to him as well. I knew how terrible he felt about me being treated in this psychiatric facility and now I was 'pulling this trick on him' as well. At that moment I really felt that I was to blame for all of this, that I was doing this to my parents, and that I was a bad kid. It didn't even occur to me, not for one second, that it could be the other way around.

After what felt like an eternity, the decision was made that I was indeed not going home with them, but that I needed to stay in the clinic for a while, to protect me from myself. And so it happened that my parents went home and left me there without an explanation. That night my Dad dropped off a bag of clothes for me and that was that. I didn't see him for quite a while after that evening.

There was a slight problem however. I was 16 years old, an adolescent, but the ward for adolescents was full. They were looking for a place in the region where they could accommodate me, but in the end I was taken to the children's ward.

I was very confused (and afraid too I guess). I did say that I would rather die than go back home with my parents, yet now my worst nightmare seemed to have become true: my parents didn't love me, they didn't care about me and they had left me here forever. Even though I really didn't want to go home, this wasn't exactly what I had planned. It was scary, especially as no one explained anything to me - not why I was there, not for how long... nothing.

I was scared and confused and that made me really restless. This caused a lot of fear in the little children on the ward, so that same evening the staff decided to put me in a small room they called the 'soothing room'.

55

Now, as a grown-up, I realise that this 'soothing room' was nothing less than a 'seclusion room' for kids. The only difference was that there was a huge mural of Miffy on the wall. Miffy is a world-famous rabbit, created by Dick Bruna. In Dutch it is called Nijntje. The image on the wall was the image that is seen most commonly: Miffy wearing her orange dress and holding the yellow bear under her arm. In theory, there is nothing wrong with this image of course.

But something went really wrong with me. I was scared and confused and my head started to do weird things. I started to see the eyes of the Miffy mural light up in red, laser beam kind of Devil eyes. With a low male voice (not fitting the cute Dick Bruna Miffy) it demanded that I pray a certain prayer out loud a 1000 times. Even though I was really scared, I started to do so, but I lost count over and over and so I had to start again and again. I was so exhausted in the end that I stopped praying, but this Conijntje (as I called the voice) wouldn't take no for an answer. He got more demanding and started to yell. I tried my best to avoid him and sat down with my face turned to the other wall, away from the mural. I hoped that if I could no longer see him, he would stop. But he didn't.

I could no longer escape or hide from this Conijntje. He wasn't just a Dick Bruna Miffy mural anymore, there was also some kind of live version of my Conijntje voice in the room; it was following me around and made sure that I would not be able to look away from his 'Devil's eyes' (in other words, besides hearing the Conijntje's voice, I also started to see a huge rabbit). He always stood where I could see him and would shout his commands at me. I had to pray, I had to hurt myself and so on. So I started to bang my head against the wall, hoping that I would no longer see or hear him. But that didn't happen. Conijntje apparently loved the fact that I was banging my head against the wall, as he was encouraging me aggressively to continue to do so.

This went on for days. Every now and again they let me out of the room, to eat and drink, to use the toilet or to take a shower. But as soon as I was outside of this room, I felt the threat of having to go back to that room (and to Conijntje), so I tried to warn the staff about this rabbit.

But as soon as I started to tell them about the rabbit, the staff immediately brought me back to the room. They probably thought I was very confused.

I spent three weeks in a row in that room. No one wanted to listen to me, or asked me what it was that I was so afraid of. That was until one particular staff member returned from holiday. He came into the room, knelt down and sat beside me on the floor. He introduced himself and asked me what it was that I was so afraid of.

At first I didn't want to answer, as so far any attempt to answer that question only resulted in me being locked up in the room again. So, what was the use of telling him? But he kept asking me and after a while I mumbled: "That rabbit", nodding my head in the direction of where I saw my Conijntje vision, which was a completely different location to where the Dick Bruna Miffy painting was on the wall.

I expected this man to stand up, to walk out of the room, and to leave me alone again but he did not. He asked me: "Would it help you if we went out of this room to talk for a bit?" The only thing I could do was to nod yes!

The same day I was 'rescued' from this room (that's really how it felt to me), I was relocated to a 'normal' room. This was still on the children's ward though. Within a week (four weeks after I entered this ward) I was ready to go 'home'.

But I didn't go home, and went to stay with a friend of the family. From there it was decided that I would be slowly working on going back home under the supervision of the clinic.

During my time on that ward, I didn't see my parents at all. I didn't see them, they didn't call, they didn't even leave me a note. Later, I was told they didn't even contact the ward to ask how I was doing and that they couldn't be reached by the staff of the ward or by the psychologists.

My leaving of the ward was not the end of my Conijntje voice. At that point, however, I didn't know this. At that moment, the Conijntje voice was gone: I couldn't hear it and I also couldn't see my Conijntje vision anymore. But I was still terrified of all the Dick Bruna Miffy images in the outside world and I can tell you from experience that the Netherlands is full of Dick Bruna Miffy images.
It seemed like no kid in the Netherlands grew up without some form of Dick Bruna's Miffy. So I guess you could say that I developed a Dick Bruna Miffy phobia. That might sound funny, but it really isn't.

On my eighteenth birthday, I was literally too old for the child and adolescent mental health clinic. It was as though by turning that page on the calendar my problems were supposed to magically disappear.

Unfortunately for me, that wasn't the case. But, as I was too old for the child and adolescent services now, I didn't get any help from them anymore.

On that last day, we as a family were due to have a last appointment with the psychiatrist. My Dad and I were the only ones to show up at this meeting. The psychiatrist told me that I was too old for child and adolescent psychiatry, but if I thought I still needed help, I could go to the local community psychiatric services.
He also told me that I should not expect too much from my life: going to university was not possible for me, living independently was a no-go also and, as to finding a job, that would be too much to ask. No, the best thing for me to do was to live a quiet life without stress. If I could do that, I might have a reasonably fulfilling life…

I never understood how this man pictured this: a life without stress. I think I am yet to meet a person who is living a completely stress free life. Yet the message this psychiatrist gave me, without blinking an eye and being very serious, was clear: life would never get any better for me. And although I no longer believe in God, I still thank God that I was already incredibly stubborn at that time.
I started a course, actually I finished two courses, I do live on my own. And yes, there were and are some problems every now and again, and there still are hurdles on my way sometimes, but I'm convinced that's just life. In terms of a job, well... that might be one area where he was right. Up until now I haven't been able to keep a regular job. I blame it on the fact that I want to be in control, that I have some authority issues and that I struggle with having a boss who tells me what to do. But I do work as much as I can, in a way that suits me.

During all these years I have seen the Conijntje vision and heard the Conijntje voice every now and again. This mostly happened while I was admitted to hospital for a time-out or around the Easter and Christmas period. I didn't understand this pattern for a very long time. The only thing I saw was the vision and voice of Conijntje and it scared the hell out of me. The fact that I was scared wasn't too bad, but by then I was hearing several voices, one of them the young Lesley and she was really terrified of Conijntje, so I had to take this into account and to work with her on this.

Around Easter 2010, I was admitted to hospital for a time-out, and it was then that Conijntje came back. I was panicking my ass off and called the psychiatrist. I do remember telling him that I didn't get it, that I couldn't understand why Conijntje was there again and why specifically at this moment. The psychiatrist told me that he had an idea: "Well, Mick, it's kind of obvious that he's back. Conijntje belongs in a clinic, that's where he appeared for the first time. You need to finally deal with your memories of that time in hospital and everything that Conijntje stands for."

That totally made sense but, back then, it was a complete revelation to me! I realised that I needed to stop giving so much power to Conijntje. He first came during my stay in the psychiatric hospital, so that was where he belonged. That was a fact, so the only way to deal with, and get rid of, the fear of Conijntje was to leave my fear at the psychiatric hospital!

The text below was written by me in my diary around Easter 2010:

Although I was terrified, that night I tried to talk to the rabbit, but it kept creeping up on me from all sides of the room. It scared the crap out of Lesley, who is the most vulnerable amongst us. When the night shift worker came into my room to check if I was sleeping, he spontaneously took the form of Conijntje (so there were actually two Conijntje 'images' in my room) and I hid behind my bed, full of fear.

This really had to stop. It's difficult to live when every living creature in front of you changes into your worst nightmare, like a 'shift shaper', and you have no clue about what is true and what is the nightmare. So something needed to change.

I spent that night thinking of a plan. The next morning I asked the staff to print off two identical outline drawings of the Dick Bruna Miffy. One was for Lesley to colour in and one was for me.

Next to my picture I wrote this text: I accept the fact that you are here, but you can no longer scare me. You no longer have any power over me. I'm an adult now and I can go where I want to, whenever I want to. I'm no longer locked up. You are just a children's book character, a fluffy bunny, nothing more. I'M IN CHARGE, I'M IN CONTROL.

The next thing I did was to write a letter to Conijntje within which I told him that the situation when he first appeared was very frightful to me. I had just told my parents that I would rather die than go back home with them and they left me there! That added just a little more anxiety to an already confused and anxious teenager.

As I kept thinking about it, I came to the conclusion that I was finally understanding Conijntje. Sometimes I thought Conijntje was my Mum: he scared me, he hurt me and he brought the worst out in me.
At other times I thought Conijntje was my Dad: fluffy and soft (sweet) on the outside, but bad with a lot of nasty, mean comments on the inside. But now, I finally knew it for sure, he was both my Mum and my Dad all in one. Conijntje played the role of both of my parents during the time they weren't there. He managed to fool me for all those years!

During my time in child psychiatry, the same thing happened as at home: I was locked up, not allowed to be part of things, put away in a small space. Conijntje told me to hurt myself and he humiliated me. That used to be the role my parents played. Conijntje took over this role. He continuously humiliated me and the abuse...well I didn't need Conijntje for that, I was doing that to myself. I selfharmed all the time.

After these discoveries, I decided, together with Lesley, to burn one of the colouredin pictures in the hospital garden. This way we could symbolically leave (the fear of) Conijntje in the hospital forever.
And although Conijntje has continued to visit me, after this time, I am way more relaxed now. I can now see Conijntje for what he is: a character from a children's book, nothing more than that.

Conijntje's image is fading and his voice is getting quieter. And me? I'm secretly smiling and feeling incredibly proud of myself. Even though not a lot of people understand, this victory can't be taken away by anyone!

Ps: I am aware that Dick Bruna's Miffy is a girl. But my Conijntje is simply a transvestite: a guy in a dress...

(Mick, May 2010)

As I wrote before, Conijntje's voice got quieter and his image faded. After a while, I thought he had gone for good... but again, he proved me wrong.
Just before Easter 2011, the Conijntje voice and image returned. So there was obviously some more work to do. This is what I wrote in my diary around May 2011:

At first, it didn't really affect me. It didn't scare me. It was only after an unexpected confrontation with some (bad) memories of my Granny, that Conijntje started to change his strategy and began to say nasty stuff about my Granny. That made it so much harder to resist letting it get under my skin. Together with some other stuff, this was the last straw - it pushed me over the edge. I started to dissociate and left to go abroad.

Once I was in a 'safe place' abroad, the Conijntje image started to change. His neck was slit and he was bleeding. He tried to talk, but there was no sound, there was only bloody air bubbles coming from his neck as he tried to speak.
This image reminded me of the memory that I have of my dog, whose neck was slit too.

Although I felt very shocked by this image, I also felt sorry for Conijntje. My child voice Lesley was so terrified that she was out of control. If I wanted to change something, or work on something, I needed to calm her down first. After that I could try to talk to Conijntje.
Lesley is terrified of Conijntje. Conijntje scares her and she thinks he's bad and scary. She is very upset, angry and sad about this.

I asked Lesley to tell me what she would do to Conijntje if there were no boundaries. So if all the bad and very mean things were allowed.

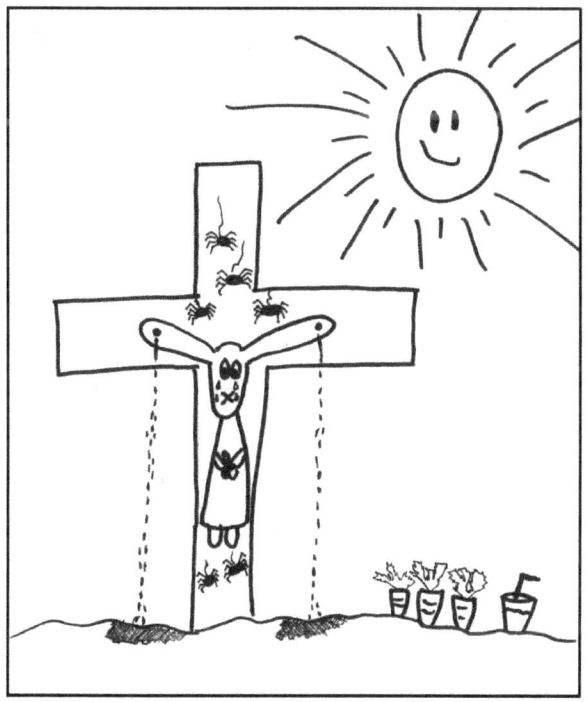

For the first time (in a very long time) I went to church to attend Easter Mass. Although I can't remember that I saw a cross with Jesus on it in there, apparently it was there. This is what Lesley told me and what I tried to draw:

"Conijntje is bad, Conijntje needs punishment. Nailed to the cross, like in church. With nails through his ears, so that it will bleed. And ropes around his hands. And spiders, because then Conijntje will be scared.
The sun is very hot. And there are carrots and cola, but Conijntje won't be able to grab them. Conijntje is crying. That's his own fault! Good for him!"

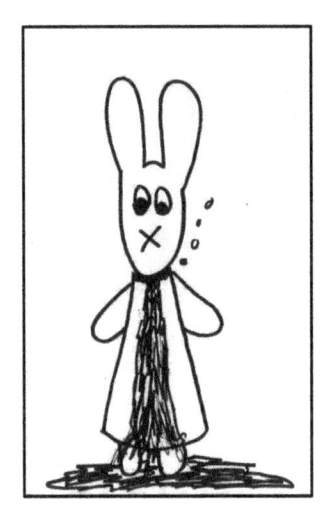

I then asked Lesley to have a good look at the Conijntje image the way he was at that moment. I asked her, "What do you see?"

This is what Lesley had to say about that: *"Conijntje is really scared. The little lights in his eyes are broken. Conijntje can't talk. Conijntje has a cut in his throat. There is blood, a lot of blood, with bubbles sometimes."*

I asked her if Conijntje was in pain. She said:

"Maybe Conijntje is in pain, but he's not crying. Crying is for girls and Conijntje is a boy rabbit.

Conijntje doesn't smile or shout or scare me anymore. Conijntje is looking very sad like dogs. Maybe we should be a bit sorry for Conijntje."

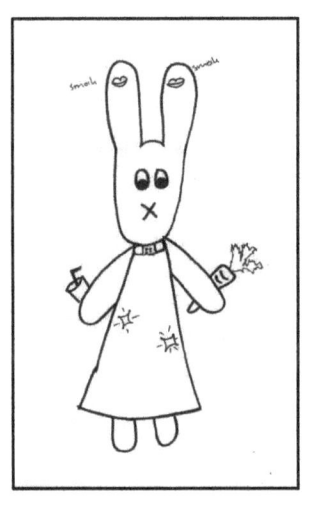

(The black stuff you can see on Conijntje's dress and on the floor is blood of course. The bubbles next to Conijntje are the bubbles coming from his airway, as he tries to speak.)

Lesley finished with saying that Conijntje might be in pain and that we could perhaps feel a bit sorry for Conijntje.

So my third question for her was: if Conijntje is indeed in pain and we might have to feel sorry for him, if you had to be nice and gentle to him, what would you do?

She answered:
"Conijntje's dress needs to be washed. It's dirty and it needs to be clean again. Conijntje will get a bandaid on the cut on his throat and no brown stingy stuff. That hurts!

And Conijntje needs a carrot and cola for when he is hungry and thirsty. He will be able to grab it for himself.

And a kiss on his ears where the nails were.

Like that, Conijntje is quite sweet, but he can't scare me any longer because it's not fun to cry. Crying tastes like the sea and stings in your eyes."

After this, Lesley was calm enough, so I could fight my own battles with Conijntje. So I decided to write to him. I wrote down what came to mind and what it made me think off. This is what I wrote:

>*There you are again, after a year of absence. I can't say that I missed you, but it wasn't so bad to see you again. I don't think you are scary anymore, if you are just there, but as soon as you start shouting and cursing and show me things that I don't want to see, then I get angry with you. And yes, that does scare me. Not so much you being there, but the things you show me. Because you are and will always be just a fluffy, cute little rabbit.*

>*I find it difficult to see you like this, with your throat slit. You remind me of my dog who was killed. Maybe that's what I'm supposed to be reminded of. I loved my dog and to see him like that was horrible. It makes me feel a deep disgust, all the way from my toes to the top of my head.*

>*That same feeling of disgust comes over me when I look at you. Not because of the image I see, but more because this should not happen to anyone, not even to you.*

What does this say about me, about you, about us?

Last year I thought that my explanation for who you are and what you represent was complete. You are my Father and Mother, all rolled into one and I 'should' hate you. But apparently I can't.

I know that in my head, I'm very preoccupied with thinking of ways to punish my parents for everything they did. And yes, in my mind I did wish them horrible things and even did horrible things to them, but only in my mind, not in real life.
But this is far out of line. No one deserves this. And maybe the solution isn't found in punishment. Maybe you punish people the most by not punishing them at all.

You disappeared, no... my fear of you disappeared when I decided to see you for what you are: nothing more, nothing less than a children's book character, a fluffy bunny.

Maybe I 'punish' my parents the most by staying true to myself and, despite everything that has happened and is still happening, by continuing to love them.

Why should we punish people at all? It will only help if afterwards they are able to see that what they have done was wrong. Only then, punishment might be useful or make sense.

If I already know upfront that it won't be of any use, why would I put all of my energy into it, into thinking about punishment in any way, shape or form?

So Conijntje, you can stop showing me those 'nasty images'. You have made your point. I've learned something. And thank you for waking me up again and keep me focused. Apparently I do need this every now and again. So, thank you.

The fact that I decided to stop thinking about a way to punish my parents doesn't mean I'm no longer angry at them or that I will hide my anger (again, like I have been used to doing my whole life). I am angry, I am furious and even that is an understatement. I'm incredibly sad, but instead of punishing them, I need to learn to cope with that anger and to find a healthy way of expressing it.

Maybe, at some point in the future I will be ready to confront my parents and to tell them what I have to say, what I think of them, and of everything that happened to and with me. But for now I don't want to waste any more energy on thinking about ways of punishing them, as that is not of any use at all. It makes me feel exhausted and it doesn't solve a single thing!
(Mick, May 14-2011)

Since that time, in 2011, I definitely said goodbye to my fear of both Conijntje and Dick Bruna's Miffy. This means that I can finally look at Dick Bruna's Miffy images, stuffed toys of Miffy, clothing with Miffy on it etc. But at the moment there is a huge sculpture of Dick Bruna's Miffy, or a person in a Miffy suit, I will get nervous again and I will feel panicky again. So far this hasn't happened, but you never know!

The fact that I can now look at images of Dick Bruna's Miffy (in the way they are meant to be seen) without freaking out, is a huge thing for me!

I would like to add a little something about the drawing I did of Conijntje, as there is a reason why I drew him the way that I drew him. In the drawing, I deliberately wounded him (cut his ear with an axe) to show that the terror image of Conijntje, with the red Devil eyes, can still be there, but the fear of him is getting less.

Conijntje is losing ground. He's damaged and he's slowly falling down and bleeding out. To me, this was a way to show that I'm finally and slowly winning my battle with him!

Sirenes
(Sirens)

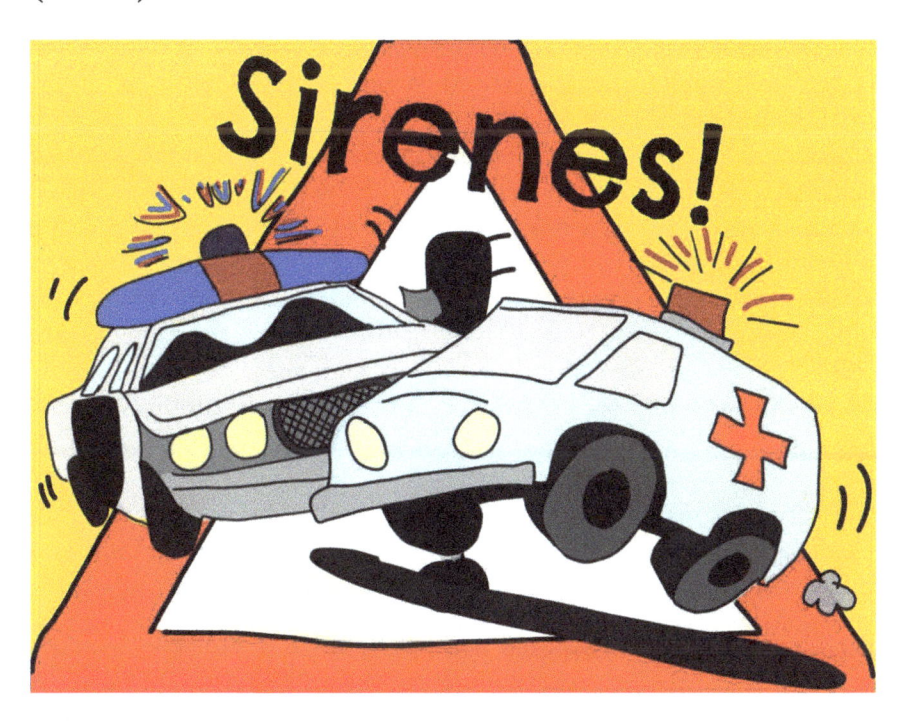

I lived next to a hospital for quite a while, so it was very normal to hear the sirens of ambulances, police cars or the fire brigade on a daily basis. There was some kind of traffic obstacle in front of my house where these cars (with their sirens on) had to wait until they could safely pass the obstacle. So the sound of sirens became kind of a normal thing for me.

When I moved to a different place in town, far from the hospital, the frequency of the sirens decreased. If I heard sirens at this time it was usually far away, or the vehicles were speeding in the streets next to my house on their way to the emergency.

I can't remember exactly when it started, but at a certain point I began to hear sirens. They were in the background, far away. But instead of fading or stopping, the sound continued. It didn't get louder, but neither did it stop. At first I wasn't very aware of the sound. It was only after a few hours that it started to make me nervous.

I searched the Internet to find information about some kind of accident or disaster that might have happened in the region. I watched both the National and local news (which I never do) but couldn't find any information on a calamity of any shape or form. Every now and again there was an ambulance passing by, just as would usually happen on a daily basis, but with these ambulances it was different as the sound increased and then decreased again. Meanwhile, in the background, I continuously heard these other sirens.

The next day, the sound got a bit louder and continued for the whole day again. My Internet, television, and newspaper search didn't give me any information on a disaster I assumed must be happening somewhere in the region. As the time went on, I became more frustrated. I couldn't deal with these sounds at this point. I was busy with other things!
I had so much to do! There were deadlines, there was work and there were so many ideas in my head that wanted to get out there into the world. At the same time I was also working on something that made me really nervous.

It still wasn't clear to me what was happening. I didn't have a clue! I started to ask a few people who I really trusted what was happening in the region. They looked at me with a puzzled look on their face, asking me what I meant. Most of the time I responded with an uncomfortable laugh and pretended that I was joking. Yet, it made me worry even more. There had to be something going on as I really did hear those sirens!

One day I directly checked it out with a friend. I asked, "Do you hear sirens too?". The answer was negative again. At first, I thought this friend might not have such good hearing, so I asked another friend, with the same result.

It slowly began to dawn on me that I might be the only person hearing these sirens. This was a very complicated thought to me. The sound of the sirens came and they went again and it took me quite a long time to figure out what was happening.

The sirens always came when there was lots of turmoil in my head, when there were lots of ideas, or when I needed to get lots of stuff done. Actually, they came at the times when I didn't have a clue about how to get everything done in time, and didn't have any idea of where to start.
The sirens started to come when I had some 'insane' weeks again. What I mean by 'insane' weeks is that I'm not very good at planning my work. So there were weeks when I had almost nothing to do, and then weeks where I would have almost had to clone myself in order to be in every place that I needed to be and to get everything done that needed to be done. I struggled to get through these kind of weeks as I had used up all of my energy long before the week had ended.

For a very long time, I wrote down when the sirens came. I also wrote down what I was doing at that point and what I still needed to do (in other words, I asked myself the question: what is going on in my life right now?) I came to the conclusion that the sirens always came when I was too busy, or had too much to do.
I like to be busy. It keeps my brain occupied, so I worry less. But when it gets too busy I feel like I'm drowning. It makes me feel overwhelmed. I feel like other people (or myself) are expecting, demanding or asking too much of me.

By now, I know that as soon as I start to hear sirens, I have to seriously take a good look at my weeks' schedule. I also need to ask myself what is going on in my life and what it is that is making me feel overwhelmed. That is what the sound of these sirens mean to me: they are my personal warning system for 'danger'! (the original purpose of sirens!)

By the way, it doesn't work so easily that the sirens immediately disappear when I adjust my weeks' schedule. I guess my brain knows me a bit better than that. The sirens start to fade away and disappear the moment it is clear that I will actually have a less busy time.

Today, the sound of sirens is no longer completely overpowering, so I can still do what needs to be done. It is now more like a kind of background noise that I don't need to focus on all the time, as I know what it means. This used to be very different, as I didn't have a clue what was going on and so could only focus on the sound of the sirens. I was convinced that somewhere in the world something had gone entirely wrong. But instead of looking at what is wrong in the world, I have now learned that I need to focus on what is wrong within me.

Unfortunately, it still works in such a way that I only realise I have already crossed my boundaries, or am too busy, when I start to hear the sirens.
I hope that one day I won't need the sirens anymore to warn me when I am about to cross, or have already crossed, my boundaries. I hope, one day, to see the overwhelm coming for myself and maybe even prevent it from happening.

Until that day comes, I'm very grateful for my internal warning system.

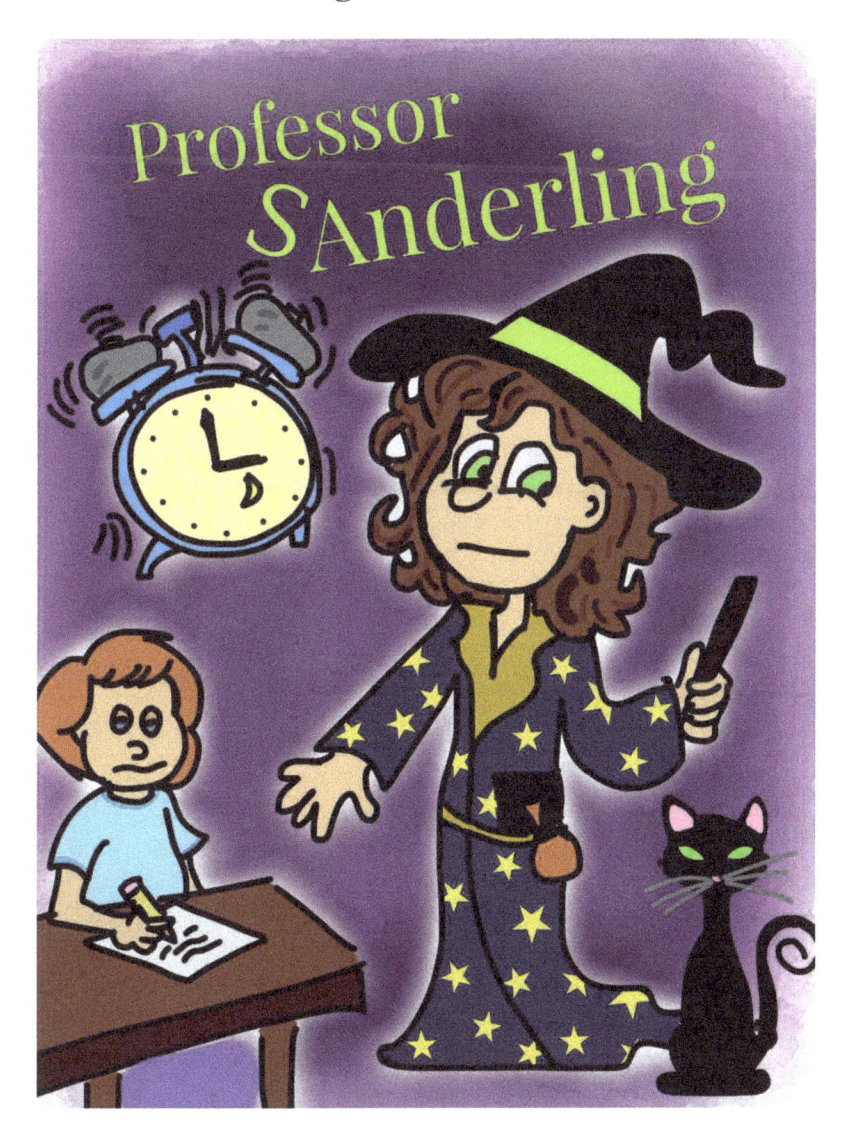

Professor Sanderling

As a kid I developed some strategies to be able to survive. My voices are just one example of these strategies. Another strategy was 'creating' my own fantasy world, which I have said something about before. This might sound as if I created both the voices and the fantasy world deliberately, but that's definitely not the case. It happened automatically, just like breathing.

When I, as an adult, try to look back at that time and at my strategies, I reason that the 'real world' was so unpredictable and threatening to me that I found it really complicated to cope with. In those days, it felt as though I couldn't influence or have control over anything. By creating my own world(s), I got some control over (at least) these worlds.

As a young kid I had already created my own world. For example: I was some kind of radio journalist and was having long interviews with others (in my head) about all sorts of subjects. I was both the interviewer and the one being interviewed in these little 'games'. I spent several hours in this way and it gave me a sense of calm and security. I was the one who made up the subjects, knew what questions were about to be asked, and also what answers were to be expected. So it was all very predictable and that made me feel calm.

A bit later in life, my fantasy world became the world of 'Ciske de Rat'. This is based on the books by the Dutch author Piet Bakker. These books are about a little boy in Amsterdam who was raised by a Mother who wasn't very interested in him. His Dad was a sailor and was hardly ever around, so he was basically on his own on the streets. Just like Ciske in the story, I also had all kind of adventures. And just as it was in this fantasy world, the fact that I was in control and decided everything was very important. I knew what was going to happen and how it was going to end. So, again, very predictable and therefore very safe to me.

You might expect that if someone is growing up in difficult circumstances and wants to escape by making up a fantasy world and various stories, this world and these stories would be all nice, happy and positive. You might expect that only happy and positive things would happen. But in my fantasy world that was definitely not the case. A lot of nasty things happened, more nasty things than positive things. To me it wasn't so much about the positive side, it was all about being in control over a very unpredictable (and therefore incomprehensible) world. So it didn't really matter what happened, as long as I was in control. I think that because there was a lot of nasty stuff going on in my real life, I tried to deal with this by using it in my fantasy world. The nasty stuff was all I knew in those years, so it was also the only stuff I knew how to cope with. I also think that I used my fantasy world to try to tell people around me what was going on in my real world. It was like a kind of 'cry for help' without having to tell them directly what was going on in my real world.

I now understand as an adult why my choice of 'Ciske de Rat' as my hero and role model made complete sense. Ciske was a little boy who grew up in a very difficult and hostile environment. His Mum abused him, locked him up and treated him like he was a piece of shit. His Dad was hardly around, so he was basically on his own. He acted out, got in trouble a lot, but is actually very gentle, caring and has a heart of gold. In a flash of rage, in one of the books, he kills his Mum, but struggles with feelings of guilt about this for the rest of his life.

The life of this little boy had so many similarities to my own life. Back then, however, I didn't see that.

When I got older, my fantasy world started to change again. 'Ciske de Rat' would be my hero for ever, but I also found another hero and role model: Harry Potter from the J.K. Rowling books. I read and re-read the books over and over again. Later on, I watched the movies repeatedly and could lose myself entirely in these stories.

In the moments when my real life started to get too chaotic, too unpredictable and therefore too unsafe, I became very confused. So I tried to make sense of my world again by stepping into my Harry Potter world. I can't remember if this was a conscious choice. To me it felt, and still feels like, something that just happened. If I can't make any sense of the world around me, I grab my Harry Potter books, or watch the movies, and it takes me to my Harry Potter world. Yet, I don't start reading the books with the intention of ending up in my Harry Potter world. I think reading these books is a soothing thing for me, just like (young) children grab their stuffed toy as soon as they need reassurance. They grab their toy, I grab these books (and my toy), even though I know it can (and will) get me into trouble.

Somewhere deep inside I felt like I was Harry Potter even though I also knew, deep down, that this could not be true. Just like the life of 'Ciske de Rat', Harry Potter's life had some similarities to my own. Until Harry left for Hogwarts, he lived at his Uncle and Aunt's house in the cupboard under the stairs and wasn't treated very respectfully by them at all.

Not only did I know for sure (on one level) that I was Harry Potter, in the moments when my world felt unsafe everyone important to me in my real world was given a part in my Harry Potter world. For example, I gave my psychiatrist the role of Dumbledore, the Headmaster. My psychiatric nurse became Professor McGonagall, Harry's Head of Department. My Mother had the part of Voldemort, Harry's biggest enemy and my Dad was given the role of Professor Snape, a questionable teacher: I kept asking myself 'is he a good guy or a bad guy?'
Nowadays, I can explain why each person got these specific roles, but back then I didn't put that much thought into it, it just happened and it seemed to feel right.

The 'choice' for this Harry Potter world is not so weird to me anymore and even makes sense. Again, there were similarities between my world and that of Harry Potter. Yet, what was even more important in my eyes, was that, in Harry Potter's world, you could solve everything that was difficult or complicated through the use of magic. There was a solution for everything in the form of a spell. For me, someone who loves magical thinking, this was a very predictable and safe idea indeed.

In 2007, I had to go abroad for a huge project. During that time, I had lots of stuff to do and my head was filled with ideas of even more things I could do. However, because of the amount of ideas in my head and the lack of time to make those ideas happen, none of my ideas made it 'out there' into the world. So the chaos in my head grew bigger and bigger. There was so much going on inside my mind that I had no idea where to start, so I didn't start at all. I kind of froze.

While I was abroad for this project, I was woken up around 3am one night. I heard a firm, but not unfriendly, female voice. It told me: "Get up Potter, time to work." I thought it was part of a dream, so I closed my eyes again, but the voice repeated in an even firmer voice: "Come on Potter, time to work, now!"
By the time I got out of bed and reassured myself there was no one else in my room, the voice came again and said: "Grab a pencil and paper Potter, we must start to work."
Although I didn't have a clue where this was heading, I did what the voice told me to do and got out a pencil and paper.

The next thing that happened was some kind of dictation, where I literally wrote down what the voice dictated to me. After a while she said: "Nice work Potter!". Then she went and I could go back to sleep.
The next morning I had a glimpse of the notes that were beside my bed. I could see some of my ideas written down in keywords and half

sentences. These keywords and half sentences meant that I was able to write my ideas down in full sentences. In this way, my ideas got out of my head and the chaos slowly reduced.

Those dictations literally gave me the space and peace in my head to be able to function during the day. When I asked the voice what her name was, she told me: "You must be kidding Potter, I'm 'Professor Sanderling' (which is the adapted, due to possible Copyright, translated Dutch name of Professor McGonagall), you know that damn well!" She didn't leave any space for arguing or any questions.

The disadvantage was that during the period when she came to help me, I wasn't sleeping very well. She only came during the moments when I had finally fallen asleep and she woke me up! Therefore, one night I asked her if we could do these lessons (as she called them) during the daytime as I might feel much fitter. I also told her that I really wanted to sleep during the night. Her answer was very short and very firm: "During the night we are the most productive, Potter!" And that was that - she kept waking me up to work.

There was another trigger for this voice. This one is not too hard to understand if you have ever read a Harry Potter book or seen a Harry Potter movie. During this time I had a neighbour who was living in the apartment next to me with his girlfriend and a cat. His kitchen was next to my bedroom.

During the night my neighbour kept the cat in his kitchen. So it happened several times that the cat, on the other side of the very thin wall, started to do what cats do: meow.
This was the moment 'Professor Sanderling' would get active, given the fact that I was already asleep of course. Since I have new neighbours without a cat, this trigger has been eliminated.

For the people who are not very familiar with Harry Potter, I will explain the logic. In the books by J.K. Rowling, Professor McGonagall is able to transform herself into a black cat when necessary or desirable. So the sound of a cat is a trigger for 'Professor Sanderling' to come out and wake me up.

Although I wished many times that 'Professor Sanderling' would help me during day time instead of during the night, I'm very grateful for her help.

Nowadays 'Professor Sanderling' is not around so often. This has to do with the fact that I haven't got so much work anymore and that I'm busy in other ways. I'm also better able to get ideas from my head onto paper or even to put these ideas into action. The chaos, therefore, does not grow so much, at least not on account of the amount of ideas.
'Professor Sanderling' only visits me now at those moments when there are, again, too many ideas in my head and I don't know where to start with them. These ideas don't have to be related to work anymore these days, they can also be about a growing 'To Do list' in my head. 'Professor Sanderling' will come when I do not know how to begin to tackle the list of things I have to do.
During the writing of this book, she visited quite regularly!

This voice is literally a helper for me that aids me in getting started with things when chaos is building up inside my head. She supports me in emptying my head (or making it at least a bit emptier) whilst helping me to put my ideas and plans into action.

Just to be clear: this voice has nothing to do with my former psychiatric nurse who, in my fantasy world, played the role of Professor McGonagall. The role of my psychiatric nurse and the role of the voice are unrelated.

Ome Jos
('Uncle Jos')

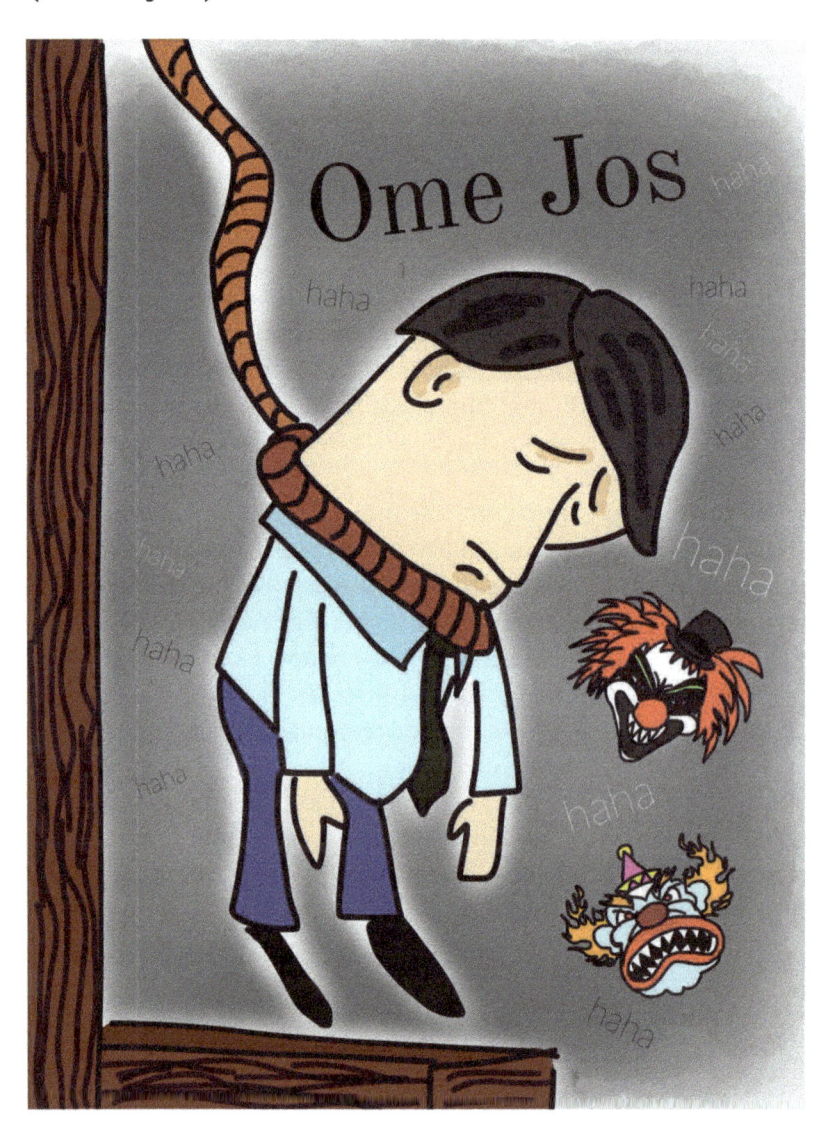

I always felt 'different', even within my own family.
On my Mother's side of the family I experienced this a bit less than on my Father's side. On the outside I might look like some of my family members, but when it comes to interests, ways of being and thinking, I am, and feel, entirely different.

When my family came together, they were always talking. Everyone would talk at the same time, without listening to one another. Everyone always had an opinion on everything, even if they didn't have a clue about the subject (but that is something I discovered later on in life). I found this really hard to cope with.

When the family gathered, to my ears and eyes there was always a lot of noise and a lot of hot air. It made me feel annoyed and sad at the same time.

You would usually find me either in the hallway or in another quiet corner of the house, far away from all the others, with my nose in a book. I withdrew to my book world and intensely enjoyed the peace and quiet I found in these books.

Yet no one really wanted me to have this peace and quiet. Every few minutes, some relative or another would find me and attempt to drag me back into the living room. I never wanted to go back so I stayed where I was. Even if I had long since finished my book, I would stay there and use my imagination to kill the time.

If I was really fed up with their whining and complaining, I would follow them into the living room. It was full of cigarette smoke and the alcohol was extensively flowing. While laughing and shouting very loudly, I had to listen to their speeches about how boring I was. I had to listen to how I "didn't belong to them, wasn't part of the family, wasn't a 'real' one". Although listening to how boring they thought I was did hurt me, not "being one of the family" to my ears sounded like a huge compliment. I didn't want to be one of them!

All these opinions, all the racism, all the looking down on and talking negatively about everyone who was the slightest bit different to how they thought they were, it disgusted me. So not being like them, in my eyes, was a good thing. But it also made me very lonely.

I don't smoke, I don't drink. I also have asthma. The cigarette smoke didn't make it any easier to stay in the same room as them. On top of that, the family would get louder and louder with every drop of alcohol they consumed and they behaved as though it made them know even more about everyone and everything. So the 'bullshit' level kept rising as well. After a few minutes, I would sneak out and go back to my quiet area. With some luck, they wouldn't notice my disappearance for the next hour. Then the whole cycle of trying to get me to come back into the room would repeat itself.

Alcohol was quite a problem within my family. As a family, one can complain and whine about others who are less fortunate in society than they are, but no family is perfect. Pretending that your own family is perfect, although there is a definite and clear problem, is, in my opinion, very hypocritical.

My immediate family were some kind of outsiders. We lived in a different part of the country and therefore didn't visit the rest of the family as much as was desired. Because we lived in a different part of the country, my brother and I didn't speak the local dialect shared by the rest of the family members (we were able to understand it though). That made me feel like we weren't special enough. My nieces and nephews were all good at something and that was being bragged about again and again and again. But my brother and I appeared to be very 'average' compared to them, so they never said anything special about the two of us.

There was, however, another nuclear family within the extended family who were considered to be outsiders. My Uncle and Aunt were both alcoholics and, because of that, they were not treated very nicely. Of course, the fact that my Aunt started to drink was blamed on my Uncle (he married into the family). He was blamed for the fact that my Aunt became an alcoholic - any other explanation was not viewed as being possible!

Every time there was a party coming up, the same questions rose again and again: how much alcohol will we buy? What alcohol will we buy? (as my Uncle drank a particular kind of booze) and (even worse) can we find an excuse not to invite them?

Every time, my Uncle was treated like the black sheep of the family. He made my Aunt drink (according to the rest of the family), he changed the atmosphere in a negative way (which, in a way, was true) and, in sum, he caused all of the problems in the world.

I did not have a very good relationship with this Uncle. When it came to taking the mickey out of me against the rest of the family, he was the first in line. He knew how to get under my skin by saying very painful and mean things in a way the others thought was very funny. So the rest of the family joined in with the laughter without realising how much his 'jokes' hurt me. And my Uncle, he laughed the loudest!

My Uncle knew exactly what to say in order to get under my skin. I really disliked him, yet not because of his drinking, as in my opinion he wasn't any worse than the rest of the family. (He might have been the black sheep of the family, according to the family, but some family members were not as 'white' as they claimed to be.)

I disliked him because he always succeeded in making me feel even smaller, more lonely and more alienated than I already was. I never 'defended' myself, never spoke back. I listened and swallowed everything I thought and felt while thinking, "He doesn't know any better".

But at some point I had enough and things changed. I was fed up with being the target of my Uncle's bullying. So I started to talk back to him and to be a bit of a smart ass, just like him. He didn't like that very much. More and more regularly I became the reason he left the party drunk and in anger, with or without the car.
My Aunt was left behind in tears. She needed to get home somehow but no one could take her as they all were drunk or had been drinking, except for some younger nephews and nieces and myself, but we didn't have a driver's license and when I did have one, I refused to do it.
Besides all of this, the atmosphere was ruined and my Aunt was at risk for getting a beating as soon as she returned home. The family blamed me for this. It was all my fault and I should have been the wiser one and kept my mouth shut. But I was fed up with being my Uncle's target and being insulted and bullied all the time. I had decided that I was no longer going to be silent.

If I'm really honest I have to admit that the times when my Uncle left with his drunk, angry head on his shoulders, it felt like victory to me. It felt like a victory over the situation and also a victory, personally, for myself.

My Aunt and Uncle's family were a kind of a mystery within the family. No one really knew what was going on within the four walls of their house. They didn't let anyone in for quite some time, and the landline had been disconnected a long time ago. So, every now and again, someone drove past their favourite pub to see if they were still visiting there. They also drove past my cousin's school to see if he was still there and how he looked (to check if he had clean clothes and so on).

There was more going on behind the walls of their house than the family could have ever imagined. This became painfully clear in 2004.

My Dad received a phone call with the announcement that my Uncle had taken his own life. He had hanged himself in the house and my Aunt had found him. So all of us (apart from my Aunt and cousin) gathered in my Grandmother's house to do the thing we were collectively best at: judging.

Everyone was in shock. How could he do this? How could he have been so selfish? How could he do this to us, to my Aunt and to my cousin (in this particular order)? There was a lot of talk about how people who took their own lives were losers, were weak, and so on.
As I was struggling myself with the question of whether I wanted to live or not, wondering whether I was going to take my own life or not, I didn't really have an opinion on what my Uncle did. My biggest question was: what was so bad in his life that made him do this? If I had learned one thing from my own struggle over time, it was that things like this are never an easy decision and are not usually made overnight. I was very sure he did not do it 'to hurt us'. My Uncle must have been in deep trouble without any of us knowing about it. Such deep trouble that he could not think of any other way out of it. To me, that much was very clear. Yet the rest of the family could not see that (yet).

The night after my Uncle's death, I started to hear his voice. It sounded exactly as he did while he was alive. Yet now he sounded kind of desperate and tried his best to be friendly with me.

He asked me to pass on a message. I had to tell my Aunt to look in a certain room, in a certain place. And I should not wait too long to tell her as it was very important.

I didn't know what to do with this information, as I thought it was a weird assignment. How on earth was I going to tell my Aunt? "Hi Aunt, Uncle is telling me to go into his room and look there and there. Oh yeah and, by the way, it's really important he says."
I could already imagine the look on the faces of my family members. They already thought I was weird, this would not make it any better. I didn't have a clue about how to do this, even if I had wanted to.

The next day, it became clear what could have been the reason for my Uncle's action. My Aunt and Uncle were due to be evicted from their home on that day. My Aunt had no idea that this was about to happen until the moment the doorbell rang. Because of this situation, she was given some extra time. I have to admit that I don't really know the ins and outs of this.

When my Dad told me what had happened, I heard my Uncle saying to me: "Do you now understand why it is so important? Hurry up!"
Even though I still didn't understand what was going on, I did understand that I had to tell my Dad in some way or another. And so I told him what I had heard.

My Dad looked at me as though I had just fallen out of the sky. It was very clear that he (just like myself) had no idea about what to do with this information. I remember saying to him: "Don't ask why, I don't know either, but maybe we should do what he says. Aunt doesn't have a lot to lose, does she?"

In the end, the solution wasn't to be found in this room, but they did find a huge stack of unopened mail, which made it clear that my Aunt and Uncle were in huge financial trouble, without my Aunt knowing anything about it. The result of not opening the mail for such a long time was a huge financial debt that could not be solved easily.

It was that bad that there was no money at all for a decent funeral. In the end, with the help of the council and some family members, it was possible to give him a funeral.

After the funeral, my Uncle's voice stayed in my head. His despair and friendliness were gone. He began to act in the way he always did to me when he was alive: arrogant, annoying and insulting.
I'm no longer afraid of him, but I do find it highly unpleasant to hear him. However, I am able to let go of the things he says about me.

To be clear, this voice is a different kind of voice from the other voices I hear. With this voice, I am convinced that he is indeed my Uncle, who is/was giving me messages. A ghost or entity you could say. The other voices represent, in some symbolical way, a problem or something that I find difficult to cope with. With my Uncle, even though his attitude changed after the funeral (back to his normal attitude I would say), I have not found anything related, in a symbolic way, to a problem in my life or something I find difficult to cope with.

To be honest, I haven't really felt tempted to have a better look at it, to see if I can find such a symbolical explanation.

I do hope that my Uncle found what he was looking for. I am proud of my Aunt and of how she is coping with life these days. She doesn't drink anymore, she has a job, she is (almost) out of debt and she lives a structured life. These are all things she could not (and was not allowed to) do while my Uncle was still alive. I realise that this might sound a bit harsh, but that's just the way it is.

Roy

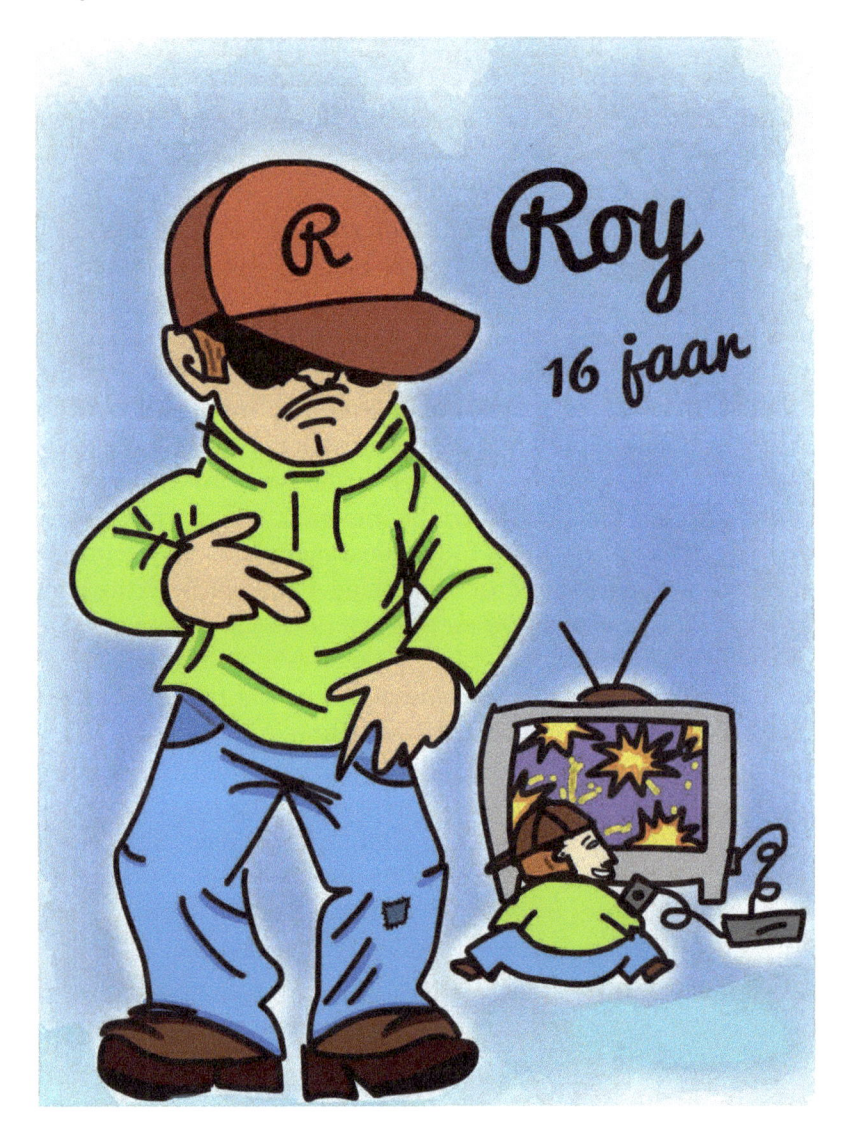

As I said before, I grew up in a violent home. The violence had many different faces: physical abuse (some even call it torture), verbal abuse (calling names, strongly or softly) and psychological abuse (giving me the silent treatment, ignoring me, belittling me etc.)

Besides all the abuse, there also wasn't any space at all to have emotions, or at least no space to show them. Within the family there was only one person who was allowed to have and show emotions and that was my Mother. But her emotions were very changeable and unpredictable. There was only one thing I could be certain of. At some point, it would end in some form of violence.

Since my Mother was the only one who was allowed to have or show emotions, it became really clear to me (unintentionally) that I was not allowed to show emotions. As soon as I showed any emotion that wasn't 'neutral', it would mean (violent) punishment. So at one point, even though I was a really young kid, I stopped showing my emotions and tried to be as neutral as possible all the time. When something like this happens for long enough, I'm convinced (by now) that a person's emotional development comes to a halt.

As a result of not being allowed to show my emotions, I didn't learn the language attached to emotions. I didn't have any words for what I felt. I didn't learn how to express myself. The feelings were definitely there, but I didn't have the vocabulary to express them. I didn't know what the emotions were called and I bottled everything up, until I exploded (usually at school, as that was a relatively safe space). Yet most of the time I didn't have any memory of these explosions. It felt as though, at these moments, that there was a big black hole in my memory. My teachers didn't believe me when I told them I didn't know what had happened. They told me that I should take responsibility for my actions, but I truly didn't know what had happened!

I had friends/voices in my head from a very young age. They were my best friends and they played games with me inside my head. By doing this, they distracted me from what was happening around me and to me. For example, if they saw a beating coming, they warned me and told me to put newspapers in my pants so I wouldn't be able to feel the beating so badly. Or if people were yelling (at me or at each other) they started to sing or to laugh really loudly, so I couldn't hear the yelling anymore.

They really helped me to survive in this unpredictable and unsafe environment. The voices didn't give me names for themselves back then, but I could tell them apart by the way they sounded and the way they said things. They were all different - different characters, different ways of speaking etc. The only thing I knew was that I had invisible friends inside my head that were always there, that were kind, that kept me company and that helped me. To me this was normal, I thought everyone had friends inside their head like me.

This changed when I was about eight years old and was walking back home from church with my best friend. I asked him how many friends he had inside his head. He looked at me with a puzzled look on his face, so I told him about the friends inside my head and repeated my question. He stopped walking, looked at me with big eyes full of fear and ran away. After this day he never wanted to play with me again and I understood that it was best not to tell anyone about my invisible friends ever again. So, that was what I did for the next fifteen years: I didn't tell anyone about them.

One of the things I learnt at an early age (and I'm not sure if I can call it 'learning') was to make myself 'disappear' in threatening or painful situations. The time when my Mum was trying to break my arm with a bench-screw, I both was and wasn't present. My body was there and was being abused, but I felt as though I was watching that body from a little distance, as a spectator. I could see what was happening, but I didn't feel it. I was like 'a fly on the wall': something is there and witnesses what happens, but rarely is part of these things or feels them.

If there was ever a fight or a loud argument at school, at home or on the streets and I felt overwhelmed by it, the same thing happened to me. My body was still there, but I had already checked out.

During those days I never really thought about what was happening. To me it was just the way it was. To be honest, I didn't really have the time to think about it. I had to be alert and was way too busy with just surviving.

The violence kept going on and on throughout my whole childhood. In some ways it is still going on today, but now I choose not to be part of it anymore, to have as little contact as possible.

As I have written, when I was fifteen years old I ended up as an outpatient in a child and adolescent psychiatric care unit. At the age of sixteen I was admitted. To me, it felt as though my life stopped at the age of sixteen. I didn't realise that actually my life started at sixteen.

When I was sixteen, just before I was admitted, I did something that was very out of character for me. I was punished for something (I can't remember what it was). My Mum told my Dad to give me a beating with an object of (my) choice. This happened every now and again, that they let me pick out my own punishment object such as a belt, a wooden shoe, a hammer or a wrench. I always picked the wrench, as that hurt the most and I wanted to show them that I was tough. Since I could 'switch off', even the strongest object was unable to hurt me as much as they might have expected it to. It was a victory for me amidst their incredible power in the situation. It did hurt though! Yet I couldn't feel that myself, so I didn't show any signs of pain.

But this day things turned out just a little bit differently. I chose the wrench but apparently didn't 'make' myself disappear soon enough and felt the first blow my Dad gave me. I can't remember what exactly happened to me, or what I was thinking, but instead of undergoing my punishment passively, I turned around and hit my Dad in the face with my fist. And it didn't stop with one punch from me.
This was the very first time I had resisted, that I had hit back. It was also the last time my Dad physically abused me.

Shortly after this, I was admitted as an inpatient. As I have mentioned previously, during a family session I announced that I would rather die than go back home with my parents. To the professionals this was a sign that I needed to be kept there, though I was never able to tell them what was really happening at home.

Emotions are still very difficult for me, this hasn't really changed. Especially anger. This has remained a 'forbidden emotion'. I continued to struggle to recognise anger for a long time and still had these 'explosions' I could not remember afterwards.

In 2012, I was working with two colleagues in German-speaking countries. We were giving workshops on a different approach to supporting people who hear voices. My experiences were used as starting point and as an example to introduce this different approach. My colleagues don't have any personal experience with voice hearing, but they had come across it during their work.
However, I got frustrated a lot with them and many times I left early, which I shall tell you more about later.

I can't remember the exact cause, but after one of these workshops things got out of control while I was in my hotel room. My colleagues heard some noises coming out of my room. When they knocked on my door and I didn't answer, they decided to come in anyway. They found me sitting on the floor, back against the wall, banging my head against the wall. By that time I already had a hole in my head and the wall was no longer white either.

My colleagues quite quickly understood that I wasn't myself. But who I was, was a mystery to them. My colleague (who speaks both German and English, but no Dutch) tried to talk to the voice that was active within me at that certain moment. The only thing that was clear was that this voice was sixteen years old and incredibly angry! But why he was angry was not clear (due to the language gap). The voice only spoke a few words of English, the rest was Dutch.

My colleague, who is used to talking to voices, did find out the voice's name -it was Roy. He also found out that Roy was really angry. But that was all. When my colleague told me the next day what had happened, I became scared. I did not know Roy yet and, for some reason, I felt very scared to try to talk to him.
By this point, I had learnt how to talk to (new) voices, but certainly those first conversations were never much fun. It was quite complicated as it tends to take time for a person and their voices to find a 'mutual language' they both can understand. I always had to get used to the way a new voice spoke - their choice of words, the way they tried to get their message across - as they all have a different manner of doing so.

It took me quite a while to finally find the courage to listen to Roy and to start a conversation with him. It took me even longer to understand who he was and his role in my life.

Roy told me that he was one of the voices I had already heard as a kid. He also told me that these childhood voices never really left me, but had just kept silent. I asked him whether there were still more childhood voices like him and, if so, why they weren't saying anything. He answered that this was indeed the case. There were other childhood voices and they would start speaking when it was their time.

Over the years, Roy told me that he used to be the one who received the (mainly physical) aggression. He was the one who took over my body while I was being physically abused, or when there was a threat of aggression around me. He literally took the beatings.
He was also the one who was there during my aggressive explosions and dished out the punches. At those moments, he also took over my body and mind. This was the reason I had these 'black holes' in my memory. When it came to these beatings I had no memory of them at all.

This is the way Roy tried to protect me from the worst aggression, but he could not always fully protect me, and he was very sorry about that.

Roy is a very cool dude. He is sixteen years old, so incredibly grown up, (according to himself). He hates it when people call him a 'kid'. He talks like a very wise teenager and behaves (sometimes) like a (less) wise teenager. But I have to admit that he is calming down a bit lately.

Roy loves computer games, and he also likes to 'make things better'. In addition to his explosive side, there is also a very caring side to him. He takes very good care of Lesley. He is very protective of her, even though he sometimes gets really annoyed with her. She really drives him up the wall sometimes! For a very long time he took on the care for Lesley in the moments when I was no longer capable of keeping calm and taking care of her. He tried to teach her how to read and write for a while. His idea was that if Lesley could do these things, she would be able to do more for herself and that would benefit all of us and make our lives easier, too.

Unfortunately, Roy didn't have enough patience to teach Lesley this stuff. When he was fed up with her, he started to be 'mean' to her. For example, he would ask her what word she would like to learn to write. Lesley would say: "Butterfly" and he would write down: 'I am a pain in the ass' for her to copy and practice. So Lesley started to practice very hard, not having a clue what she was writing. After I had a firm talk with him, Roy quit his efforts and another (adult) voice took over the responsibility for Lesley, so Roy could be a teenager again. But he still takes care of her, in his own special way.
Another thing that became clear to me is that Roy, up until a year ago, was still taking care of the aggression and anger side of things. He continued to express my anger for me. He also continued to protect me from the anger and aggression of others. Although he meant well, it didn't really help me. It made it difficult for me to learn how to express anger for myself, or to cope with other people's anger. This was what I wanted, to be able to experience and express anger for myself.

In 2014, I attended my first 'Be the Change' workshop. To those of you who don't know what this is, it's a workshop designed by the founders and creators* of the American concept, 'Challenge Day'.

Challenge Day was developed to show children in High Schools that they had more in common than they thought. The idea was to show them that they aren't so different from each other. And if you are not so different from each other, why bully each other? You could call it an anti-bullying program, but it's way more than that. It's also a leadership program. 'Be The Change' workshops are the equivalent of Challenge Day for adults.

During these 'Be The Change' workshops one can do some 'anger work' to let go of all the anger inside in a safe way.

I skipped this part during my first workshop as I was scared that Roy would take over and beat the shit out of the other people. That would definitely not be acceptable, nor something that I would want to happen. During my second workshop I made a deal with Roy. I asked him if he could let me practice with anger by myself, without him interfering. I told him that I would really appreciate it if he gave me the opportunity to practice by myself. So it happened that, for the very first time in my life, I could scream and yell and be angry as myself. I can tell you from experience, it is exhausting.

Late that night, the usually cool and energetic Roy was as quiet as a mouse. I decided to have a talk with him.

I: What is going on, you are so quiet?
R: ......(with a very tiny, sad voice) Do I need to go now?
I: What do you mean? Why do you think you need to go?
R: (sobbing) Well, you demonstrated today that you can be angry yourself, that you are very good at it. But that was my job. And if you can do it yourself, then there is nothing left for me to do.
I: I don't want you to go, I'm very happy with you. But I do want to learn how to be angry and how to cope with the anger of others for myself, that is true. But that doesn't mean I want you to go. Maybe we can think of something else for you to do? There are lots of things that I need a little help with.
R: But I'm not good at anything else...
I: That's not true at all, I know something that you are very good at, and I'm not!
R: What is it?
I: Well, when it comes to expressing and coping with anger, I'm a newbie and you are a pro. Maybe you want to become my anger coach?
R: Yeah cool! Then you will always have to listen to me!
I: I hear you, but that is not what a coach does. A coach will give advice and then lets the person try for himself. Afterwards, he can tell the person how he did - what was good and what could have been done differently. It

doesn't mean that I always have to do what you say. I need a chance to practise and to make my own mistakes, so I can learn from those mistakes. You do things your way and I need to find my way. I should not turn into a copy of you. Do you understand?
R: I do understand, but then you will never listen to me and will only do the things you want to do!
I: That is definitely not my intention. If you have good advice for me, I will certainly consider it and try to use it. What do you think? Shall we just give it a go for a while?
R: …… OK.
I: Deal?
R: Deal!

So now, Roy is my anger coach. And we are both improving in our new roles. In the beginning, Roy still took over a bit too quickly when I became angry, or when there was aggression around me. Yet now he's giving me more and more space to practice and will always politely ask me if I want him to step in and take charge of a situation. He lets me try and afterwards gives me advice on what could have been done differently (or 'better' as he would put it). I have to say, I really like it this way of doing things. And he does too.

If you were to ask me what Roy represents, what his job is, I would say that he is there to teach me how to cope with (and express) both other people's anger, rage and aggression and my own.

Why do I think that he is sixteen years old, and stays sixteen years old, even though I age?

Roy told me that during my childhood he was a kid and was the same age as myself. Every birthday that I had, he grew older with me. I had asked the childhood voices at the age of twelve to please go away and leave me alone, as I wanted to be a normal teenager in school instead of the freak my fellow students thought I was for talking out loud to my (invisible) voices. They didn't go away, they just kept silent for many years, but they were still there.

At the age of sixteen, it was a very significant moment when I hit my Father back for the very first (and last) time. That was the very first time Roy and I were there simultaneously. That's where he got stuck in age, as things from then on started to change.

* founders Challenge Day: Yvonne and Rich Dutra-St John.
website: www.challengeday.org

Rik
(The text on his shirt says: 'Girls are STUPID!')

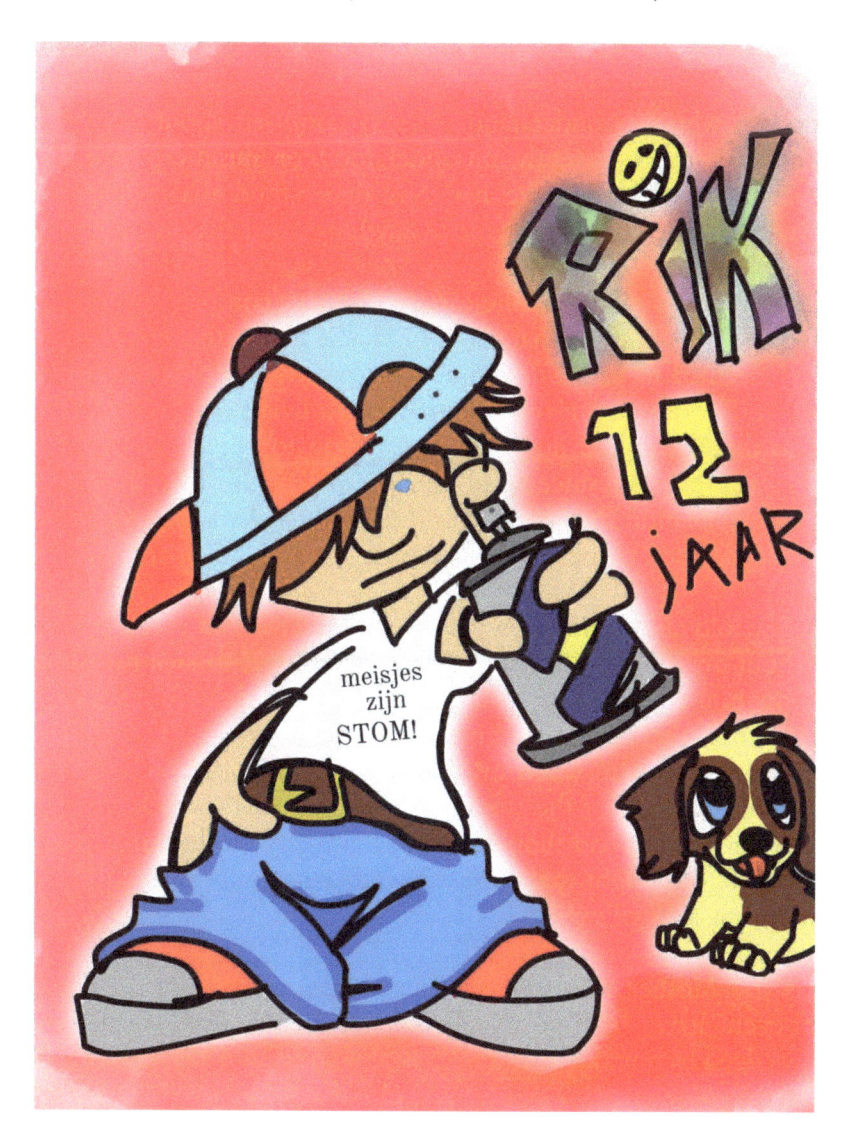

I was born as a twin. But my twin brother unfortunately didn't make it. He was stillborn and the doctors explained to my parents that I used all of the nutrition. There was not enough left for him to fully develop.

My mother, who was understandably very confused about what had happened to her, apparently misunderstood or misinterpreted the information the doctors gave her. She understood that I 'ate' my brother and so she couldn't see me as anything other than really evil.

My Mother is very religious. She can also be very confused from time to time. She doesn't think that she is God, she is sure that she is God! My birth seemed to prove this to her, as only God decides about life and death. She had just given birth to both a living child and a dead child, so there could be no other explanation to her aside that she, herself, was God. And since I had 'eaten/killed' my brother, there was no other explanation than that I was the Devil. As I was still a child, I was conceptualised as the Devil's child.

I was only told about this a few years ago. My Dad had come to visit me without my Mother after an incident when I had to kick my Mum out of my house as she was behaving in a horrible way. As he visited alone, he had the chance to give me some information he would never be able to share when my Mother was around. This piece of information was one of the things he shared. For my whole life (up until that moment) I had thought that the way my Mother treated me was my fault. I thought that I must have been a really bad kid or, as she called me, a Devil's child.

I guess my Mother was really confused during that time and she might even have had postnatal psychosis, but that was never acknowledged by any doctor.

My Mother wasn't capable of taking care of me and persistently refused to do so. For that reason, my Granny came to our place from Monday to Friday to take care of me. During the weekends my Dad was at home and took care of me. My Granny would go home for the weekend to be with my Grandfather. My Mother did take care of my older brother by the way. I always remained her Devil's child. She could not see me any differently.

From a very young age I was raised as a boy, both by my Mum and my Dad. I wore my brother's old clothes, had no 'girl's toys' and was not allowed to 'act girly'. There was one exception: when family members came to visit. At these times I had to be a girl. I had to wear a dress and had to 'act girly'. I didn't understand this at all. I was very sure, there was no doubt about it, that I was a boy.
Even though I did notice that my brother had some different parts to his body, it did not make me doubt my gender, as my brother also had a different eye colour, so why couldn't a body be both different and equal at the same time? To me, this was a fact: I was a boy and nothing could change my mind about this.

When I was twelve years old, I went to High School and for the first time in my educational history I had separated sports lessons. The class was divided up into girls and boys. To my surprise, the teacher put me into the girls' group. I was sure that he had made a mistake. So I walked up to him and told him that he had made a mistake and that I had to be in the boys' section, as I was a boy.
The teacher looked at me and started to laugh out loud. He looked me in the eye and told me that I should quit goofing around, that there was no mistake and that I had to go back to the section where I belonged: the girls' section.

I was totally confused and didn't understand a single thing about it. I was a boy, yet I was being sent to the girls' section. Most of the time I was not allowed to join as I was too rough, too wild, too strong, or too boyish.

Apparently I was neither: definitely not a girl, but not a boy either. So I was 'nothing' and this made me feel very sad and lonely.

A bit later when I entered puberty (I was quite late with this) and my body started to develop, I became even more frustrated. I got breasts, but that was so wrong as I still felt as though I was a boy! So I started to bind them with really tight bandages, as tight as possible to hide them and to make them go away. But this didn't prevent those things from growing of course.

In the meantime, my Mum thought that I needed a bra and announced this to everyone around and near us. As if this wasn't embarrassing enough, she also got mad when I resisted this need for a bra. I was sure that I didn't need one. Those things just needed to disappear.

A little bit later, when I had my first period, I didn't have a clue what was happening to me. No one ever prepared me, or given me any sex education, so I had no idea what was going on. I seriously thought that something was really wrong with me and that I was going to die because of all the blood loss. The first couple of times I didn't dare to tell anyone about it and tried to help myself with (lots of) toilet paper. This monthly event felt like monthly torture. When I finally found out what was happening and what the reason for it was, it felt like further proof that something was wrong with me. Why did I have to have my period when I had no intention of having kids, not now, not ever! This period thing was completely useless! And besides that, I still didn't feel like a woman, so it didn't make any sense…

I still dressed boyish, I still liked 'boy things', I was still too rough, too active, too strong and too wild. I had short spiky hair and people started to label me a 'dyke'. To my classmates it was obvious: I was a lesbian and no other explanation existed for them. No one ever thought to ask me if what they were thinking was correct or not.

These rumours and the bullying weren't something I enjoyed very much. So I decided to let my hair grow long again. Maybe that would make me a girl. But it didn't work like that, it only made me feel even sadder and more powerless.
This feeling of 'I'm nothing, not male, not female' kept haunting me. The feeling was worse at some times than at others. Yet it never left me. It was like the ocean: it came and went in waves, sometimes severe, sometimes hardly there at all.

In July 2012, a lot was happening in my life. I had a neighbour who was causing lots of trouble. He threatened the other neighbours on a regular basis, especially me. He put me up against the wall and stood really close to me, so I had no chance of getting away. This was kind of threatening for me, as he was a really tall guy and I'm not at all tall. At moments like this I could not get away from him.
I did everything in my power to get rid of this person from our apartment block but, despite all of my efforts, it didn't work out. I felt so powerless. On the one hand there was this huge, threatening, tall neighbour and on the other hand there was the bureaucracy of my housing company!

My work (in a 'regular' job) was also quite challenging for me at this time. I felt powerless in this area of my life too and as though I wasn't being taken seriously.

Altogether, it wasn't a nice time and there was more stuff going on than my head could handle.

One of the neighbours across the street had a dog staying over for a couple of days. That dog looked almost the same as the dog we used to have at home. One day, while I was walking back from the supermarket to my home, we came across this dog and Lesley wanted to pet it. The neighbour was ok with this and Lesley was a very happy bunny.

That night I was woken up by Lesley's crying. I also felt a lot of pain in my leg. When I turned on the lights, I saw that my bed was covered in blood. When I looked at my leg I could see the word 'bitsj' (which is the English word 'bitch' spelled phonetically) carved on to my leg. That scared me a lot! I had hurt myself before, but I could not remember doing this and had never carved words on my body before. It didn't make any sense to me. I thought that Lesley was crying for the pain I felt, but this was not the case.

Next to my bed, one of her toy dogs was lying there with huge, different kinds of cuts all over its body. In the middle of a huge gap on its back there was a small kind of pitchfork driven into its body. This was the reason that Lesley was hysterical.

I was scared as there were things happening that were totally out of my control. After a telephone call with my crisis manager, we came to the conclusion that I might have a new voice which held a lot of anger inside. This was a very frightening idea to me.

This voice was Rik, a cool twelve year old boy (but emotionally much younger). Just like Roy, he was one of the voices I had during childhood. During that time he was always the same age as me, but when I reached twelve he did not get any older.

Rik was incredibly angry! He kept cursing at the 'bitsj'. His usual vocabulary consisted of: "Girls are stupid"; "We don't need any girls"; "Everything started when she became a girl".
Naive as I was, for a very long time I thought that Rik was talking about Lesley. Sometimes he was, but most of the time he wasn't.

The reason Rik abused Lesley's toy dog was that he felt jealous of Lesley. She had petted the dog and he wanted to do that too, yet Lesley was one step ahead of him. So, in revenge, he cut her dog open, as he knew that she would be devastated.

During the time that followed, a lot of things got destroyed in my house. My body was often destroyed too, and every now and again I found messages written in my own blood on my walls and floors. I did not like that and it scared me a lot.

The crisis manager and Rik had a serious conversation. Rik told my crisis manager that he didn't want to keep destroying things, he actually wanted to create things. He wanted me to be proud of him, but I never was! He wanted to comfort me and to make me happy, as he didn't like it at all when I was feeling sad. But he didn't always manage to make me happy and that frustrated him. Out of frustration he then destroyed things. Often these were the things Lesley loved as he hated her for being a girl and not just a girl, but a cry-baby girl.
As I didn't like the fact that he was writing and drawing with my blood on the floor and the walls, I decided to get him a sketchbook and some markers. This way, he could be creative in his own sketchbook. And so it happened on a regular basis that I woke up and there were lots of (beautiful) drawings waiting for me in the living room.

Sometimes the drawings were not so pretty, but, instead, very sad or very angry. Yet the drawings he made became a starting point for conversations about what was happening (with me).

Rik usually knew what was

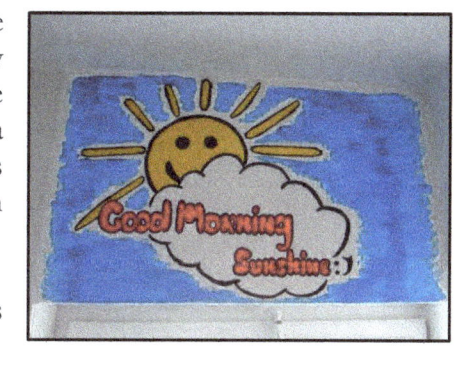

bothering me way before I knew and he tried to tell me with his drawings. In that period he was the one who told me what was happening in and around me.

So, he did not only destroy things…

One morning, after having a difficult evening, I walked into the bathroom and found a mural he had made me in the hope that it would cheer me up a bit. And he created more nice surprises like this.

Rik's main bullying target continued to be Lesley. He kept repeating the sentences: "Girls are stupid", "We don't need any girls", "Everything started when she became a girl".

Rik was very into symbolism. If he felt I wasn't listening to him, he would show me what he was trying to say. For example, he cut the ears off Lesley's toy dog, and she was devastated.
His words stayed the same. He hated girls and everything that was girly.

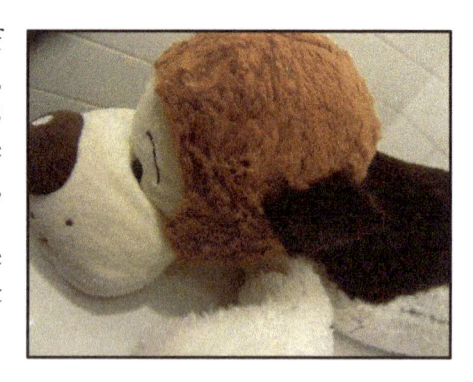

During the times when I was struggling with the question, 'What am I?' he would be incredibly silent or hyperactive, repeating his message about how bad girls were. I still didn't get it. I did know that I felt more male than female but, well, what is a person to do with that feeling?

In May 2014, as I mentioned before, I went to a three day workshop called 'Be The Change' (BTC) for the first time. I was struggling again with my eternal dilemma: 'What am I?'. During this workshop everyone is given the opportunity to share something personal about themselves with the group. This is what I had to say that day:

> "If you really knew me, you would already know more than I do, as I have no idea who I am. Even worse, I have no idea what I am. I don't feel like a woman, but I don't entirely feel like a man either. I feel like nothing. And I find that really complicated, as people keep telling me that I should just be myself. Yet how can I be myself if I don't even know what I am? It feels like I can only find out who I am after I have answered the question of what I am. This feeling of being nothing makes me feel really sad and lonely."

I did know (by now) that this feeling had a name: I was transgender. Yet to say this out loud was a huge step. I felt like a 'freak of nature' and as though I was the only one in the world who was struggling with this.

Via the BTC facilitators I was introduced to a transman* from Canada. After the BTC I emailed him quite frequently. This felt really good. I wasn't the only one! There was at least one other person in the world who knew how I felt! He was already way ahead in his process, so he could give me advice about the things I was struggling with.

So I started my first steps on this uncertain path, without a clue as to where it would lead me. Yet this path had its own momentum, as though it was unstoppable.
The first thing I did was to cut my hair short. Although that might sound really simple, it felt like such a relief to me. With my 'male haircut' (as the hairdresser called it) I felt so much more akin to something that could be myself!
If people on the street or in the supermarket looked puzzled as they had no idea about how to address me (as male or female) it felt like a small victory.

My next step was to buy a special piece of clothing to 'hide' my breasts. It's called a 'binder'. I just wanted to try it out and to experience how that would make me feel. Again, it felt like a relief and the puzzled look at other people's faces was an increasingly regular occurrence. Every time people seemed confused and got my gender 'wrong', it made me feel happier. I had never felt so much myself as I felt at this point in my life.

And Rik??? Rik was happier too, and angry less often. He kept sending messages explaining that he was glad I was a real boy again. These days, he doesn't argue with Lesley so much. As long as I'm feeling great, he's feeling great too.

Rik is able to take over and take charge. Sometimes I have no memory of it at all, but sometimes I do. At these moments, he's at the steering wheel and decides where we go, and I'm in the passenger seat and can only watch and talk to him.
When he completely takes over, he often sends emails or text messages to people I know. Rik writes phonetically, so it's quite a task to be able to read it.

Rik also loves computer games. He doesn't do a lot of drawing lately, as I am doing that myself more and more nowadays. It is just when something is going on with or in me that I don't understand that a drawing created by Rik will show up.

Rik is still there 24/7. He is still annoyed by everything that is (too) girly according to him and that will probably never change.

Rik used to be one of the child voices. During my childhood he dealt with the verbal aggression so I did not always have to endure that myself.

If you were to ask me what Rik's role is in my life, I would have to mention at least two important tasks: Rik makes me aware of my gender issues and he also makes sure that I will no longer ignore or avoid these issues.

Rik's other task is to make me aware of how and what I feel inside in those moments when I'm not able to feel things yet. In this way he is (via his drawings) also a mediator between myself and the other voices. When the other voices want to make something clear, and perhaps feel like I'm not listening closely enough, they can ask Rik to get my attention via a drawing about the issue they want to address. In this way, the issue can become part of the consulting hour and I can no longer ignore or avoid it.

Even though I don't know where my 'transgender journey' will take me, I do notice that my desires and thoughts about it keep changing. A year ago, for example, I told people around me that I didn't want to do certain things (like changing my name) as they didn't apply to me at that time. Yet now, a year later, I have taken some of those steps or am still working towards them. It's a process. By now, I know that processes are always changing and developing, even if it doesn't always seem that way. I have also learnt that the decisions within this process can only be made when I'm ready for them. So, God knows what the future has in store for me.

I'm really grateful that Rik keeps me focused regarding this gender issue, as I now feel (already) more myself than I have ever done.

* A transman is a person who was assigned female at birth but whose gender identity is that of a man.

The Polar Bear

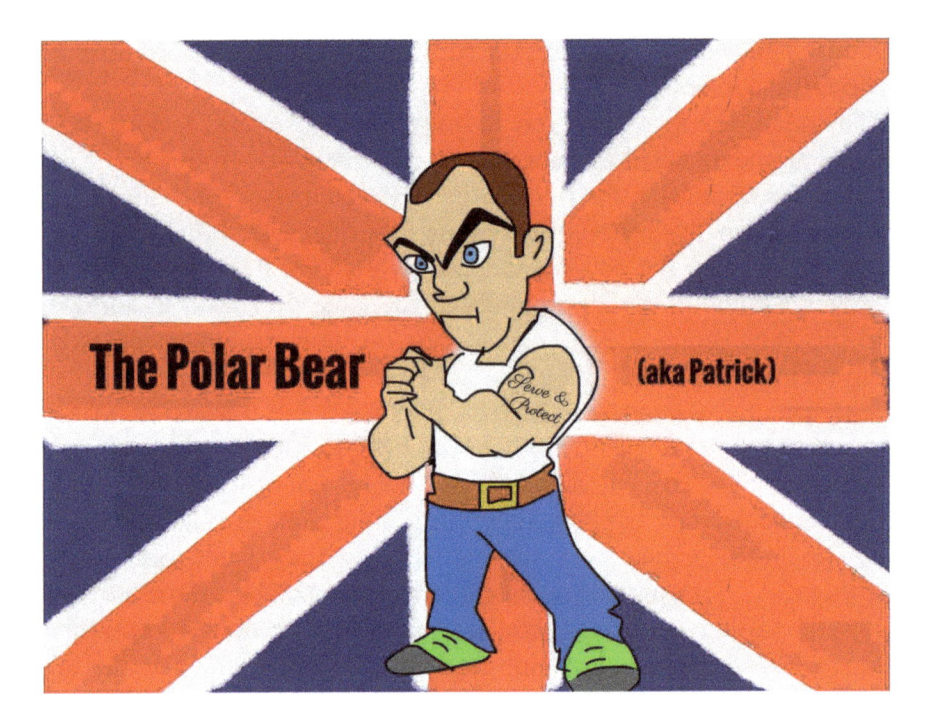

I can't remember exactly when 'The Polar Bear' came into my life. So I can't precisely tell you what was happening in my life at that time. I do know that he tells me that he has been with me my whole life, but he only started to talk to me during adulthood.

'The Polar Bear' is the exact same age as me, we share the same birthday and his official name is Patrick, but only Lesley and Rik can call him Patrick and Rik only very occasionally.

'The Polar Bear' only speaks English. He is very capable of speaking Dutch, but he prefers English. He only speaks Dutch to Lesley as she can't understand English. He is speaking more and more in English to Rik, as he thinks Rik should learn this language as soon as possible.

'The Polar Bear' is a man of few words. He takes care of 'the whole system' and he will take over if he thinks it is necessary. He takes care of Lesley in those moments when I no longer have the strength or the patience to do it myself. She sees him as her Daddy.

'The Polar Bear' only takes over when he thinks it is necessary. This is usually when I am up to 'stupid/dangerous' things (mostly hurting myself, but sometimes worse). On most occasions he will consult me, but if I don't agree he will act on his best abilities and do whatever he thinks is right in that moment.

'The Polar Bear' always informs my caregivers about what is going on by email. These emails are typically in English. He will inform them in short, clear sentences about what is going on, why he thinks he needed to take over and what kind of actions he took (for example, medication). He also lets them know when he thinks he will be able to let me return.

Here is an example of an email 'The Polar Bear' once sent:

> **Subject: to inform you.**
>
> *Just so you know: I took over.*
> *He's in so much pain that he's up to no good in order to shift the pain to a more familiar kind of pain. I won't let that happen, so I'll go to bed and make sure he's about to have a good night of sleep.*
> *I'll try to get him back tomorrow morning, but if he stays like this, I'll stay in charge till you are there.*
> PB

Everything 'The Polar Bear' does is to make sure that I'm doing ok, or that I will do ok again in the near future, kind of to protect me from myself. This can mean protecting me from self-harming, or giving me a time-out because I can't find my peace. Apparently, deep within me, I find it incredibly difficult to take good care of myself. This is one of the (many) things I still need to work on.

As I have already said, 'The Polar Bear' is the same age as me. He ages alongside me with every birthday. His name, Patrick, is not something that I came up with. He told me this himself when I asked him for his name.
His other name, 'The Polar Bear', arose during a conversation between him and my psychiatrist when he said that I had been "frantically walking up and down the room like a frickin' Polar Bear". The psychiatrist didn't understand him correctly and called him Polish Bear, but he didn't agree to that name. From that moment onwards he was 'The Polar Bear' and he felt ok with this.

If I think about who he could be, there is only one thing that comes to mind. Earlier, I talked about my birth and about being one of a twin. My twin brother was a stillborn. His name was Patrick. My second name is Patrick as well. I think 'The Polar Bear' could be my twin brother. I did ask him about this once or twice, but he neither confirms nor denies this fact. He keeps saying it's completely irrelevant and that the only important thing is that he's here.

So, I have stopped trying to figure it out. Also, to me, it is indeed the most important thing that he is here and exists in order to protect me. While I'm writing this, he's telling me: "That's right!".

If you were to ask me about 'The Polar Bear's' function, I would say that he is a helper, someone who keeps me company in moments when I'm having a difficult time and when I'm lonely. He is someone who stops me in moments when I'm suffering from my gender dysphoria and am about to adjust my body myself by destroying the parts that, according to my opinion, should not have been there in the first place.

He's also the one that makes sure I will get home safely, regardless of where I am. He's 'De Brutaalste's' best friend and is like a Daddy to Lesley as well as being a companion to her. Together with 'De Brutaalste' he keeps an eye on the others at those times when I can no longer do this myself.

I would almost say he's my guardian angel.

'The Bully Pecking Order'

Now that I have introduced the three youngest in my head, I would like to tell you a little bit more about the interactions between them. Sometimes people accuse me of making the experience of hearing voices look like a hugely happy event, like it's always nice and cosy. And even though I have never meant for it to come across like that, I do understand their criticism. The thing is, I'm only human and I prefer telling people about my successes instead of all the things that drive me insane and I can't find a solution to!

One could consider the voices in my head to be a huge family system. They function together as a family, but they can also function as individuals. Some voices are each other's best friends, whilst others can't stand each other and would be happy to kick the other out of my head. The problem is, this is not a possibility.

There are moments when there are some kind of bullying epidemics inside my head. The voices responsible for this are mainly the younger ones: Lesley, Rik and Roy.

It might be clear from the earlier chapters that Rik doesn't like girls in general, but especially the girl he can't run away from: Lesley. He really doesn't like her (in fact, he almost hates her) and usually calls her a 'fuckup'. He can't stand her, nor the fact that she is afraid of almost everything, nor the fact that she cries about almost everything. This is something Rik can't understand at all. He blames all of this on the fact that Lesley is a girl.

Lesley gets on Rik's nerves all the time and he certainly lets her know! He regularly bullies her. It is more than just teasing, as in the example I gave before about the dog on the iPad. Rather, he deliberately scares and hurts her. He teases her about her drawings and tears them up. Lesley works really hard on these and is often very proud of them.

Rik destroys her toy animals or threatens to do so. He also sabotages activities that Lesley really enjoys.

When I attempt to speak with Rik about this and ask him why he is behaving in this way -a lesson in asking deeper questions- the usual outcome is that he, for some reason, becomes very angry. Most of the time he is angry at Roy as Roy bullies him and Rik doesn't like that very much. Rik doesn't feel that he can beat Roy, so instead he projects all of his anger on to Lesley and starts bullying her because she's an 'easy target'.
Roy knows very well that Rik has a short temper and is not afraid to use that against him. Roy finds Rik's short temper very amusing. The only thing Roy needs to say to Rik, for example, is that he's acting childish or, even worse, that Rik is acting a bit like Lesley, and Rik will explode!
RIk explodes even more virulently when Roy teases him in relation to his name ("Oh gee, there is Rik, with his non existent dick! It's so little, he must be a girl!"). I think it is understandable why calling Rik a girl is the worst possible insult for him. The result is a very angry Rik who starts bullying Lesley and sometimes even destroys my stuff and my house. Things are literally being destroyed at my house on a regular basis, sometimes even very important things.

If I talk to Roy and ask him why he is doing what he is doing, it doesn't take me very long to understand that Roy is being bullied by 'De Brutaalste' and 'The Polar Bear'. Roy thinks of himself as very grown up and, as a result of this, he thinks he can solve EVERYTHING. But as soon as things don't work out the way he wants them to, or it turns out that he can't solve a problem of some kind, 'De Brutaalste' and 'The Polar Bear' will make fun of him. They think Roy is arrogant and cocky, and believe that he should get off his high horse. Yet when they try to tell him in a normal, civilised way, Roy goes into his cocky, arrogant teenager mode even more: he tries to show the two ancient gentlemen (or the dinosaurs as he often calls them) that they should not butt in and that he definitely knows what he is doing. They know it's no use of trying to talk him out of it, so they start to tease and bully him instead.

So, Roy is being bullied by the adults and takes it out on Rik. That makes Rik feel very angry, so he takes it out on Lesley. In many ways, it all operates like a normal family or even society in general. People do not usually pick a stronger, bigger victim but one they are pretty sure they can handle.

The difference between having children inside your head and having children within a regular family is that in a regular family you usually have more tools to get your kids back on the right track. This is the most frustrating thing about having these children inside my head: they can drive me insane with their behaviour!

For example, I can't pick one of the children up or send him/her off to their room, or put them on a 'naughty step'. I can threaten them as much as I like, but I can't make it happen! I can't walk away from my kids. And if I tell them no, that will be a losing threat as well. They will just take over my body and do as they please anyway. They know very well that my threats are made of nothing more than thin air and that they will get what they want in the end. So they laugh at me when I send another threat their way.

The bullying can literally drive me crazy as I have no idea about how to make it stop. These are the moments I find the hardest to cope with in relation to hearing voices. I do not have a clue about how to raise 'non-embodied' kids.

If anyone has a solution, please tell me! Even after all these years I still have no idea of what to do. Of course, there are lots of moments when they are all getting along fine, when they are very caring towards each other and stick up for one another. But in those moments when they don't, it can drive me insane!

De Moederstem
('The Mother Voice')

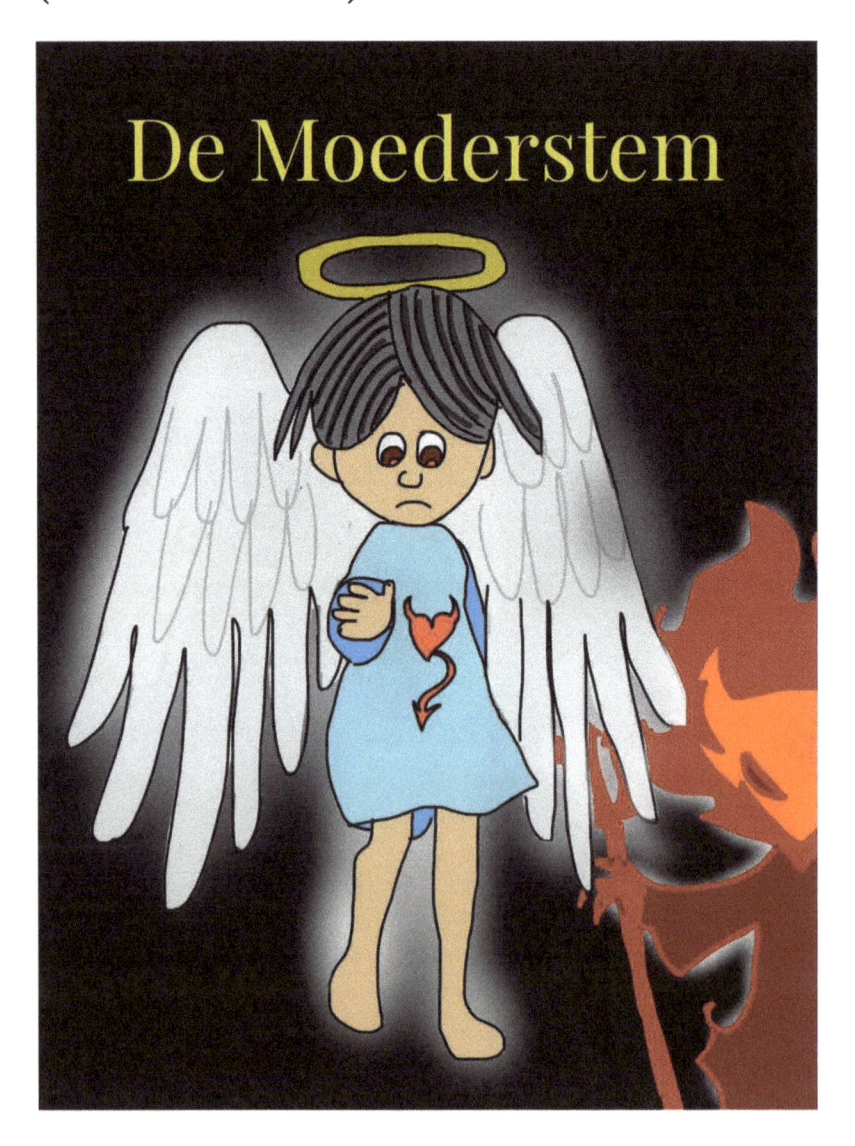

I think it might be clear by now that I don't have a very close bond with my Mum.
To me, she has always been a very unpredictable person. I could never estimate how she would be, so I never knew how to behave around her, to 'do it right'. One moment the way I behaved was ok, but within a minute her 'state of mind' (or opinion) could change 180 degrees and the same behaviour was entirely wrong. That would lead to punishment varying from being ignored to breaking my bones and all the (un)thinkable things that are between these opposites.

My Mum is very religious and from time to time, this takes on extreme forms.

Through my twin brother dying at birth (and maybe even before this) my Mum became convinced that she was God. By interpreting the words of the doctors incorrectly, she was convinced that I was the Devil or at least a Devil's child.

I was only told about my stillborn twin brother a little while ago, and that kind of sucks as this piece of information explains a lot about how I was treated (although this doesn't make it right in any way of course) and influenced my life big time in a negative way.
Now that I know this piece of information, I can understand that my Mum's behaviour towards me had nothing to do with me being an evil person and everything to do with my Mum's unprocessed grief.

My Mum could (or would) not take care of me. She took care of my older brother but she ignored me. She didn't feed me, didn't change my nappy, didn't pick me up, nothing at all. She didn't speak to me, but if she had to speak to me she addressed me with the terms, 'Fuckup' or 'Devil's child'.

My Dad had a very busy job and only came home late in the evenings. This is why my Granny came to our place from Monday to Friday, mainly to take care of me. My Dad was home at the weekends and took over my care from my Granny. This went on for the first three years of my life. After these three years, my Granny had to stay at her own home to take care of my very ill Grandpa.

From that moment, at the age of three, I was kind of on my own when it came to survival. More than this, I was also handed over to my Mum's dangerous moods.

Every time I came or was home, I had to keep my guard up. I tried to be as invisible as I could be. I was always looking out for signs that may suggest or predict how my Mum was feeling and what, therefore, was the best way to behave.
This was all very unpredictable, which made the situation impossible; there were hardly any signs to be found. What was ok now could be, without any cause, completely wrong within the next minute. This felt totally unpredictable to me and, therefore, very unsafe.

On occasion I could recognise some signals. My Mum would get this certain look in her eye, which I would call the 'Devil's eye glare'. In my memories there is some kind of little red light in her eyes at moments like these, but I now think it might have been my fear that conjured these lights up. As soon as I spotted this 'Devil's eye glare' I tried to get out of the room, but usually by then it was already too late.

As soon as my Mum got this 'Devil's eye glare' I knew trouble was on its way. These were the moments when the abuse was the worst.

When I think of these moments now, I seriously wonder if my Mum was 'present' or if she, like myself, in some way kind of dissociated*. As the adult I am today, it's very difficult to understand how and why someone can do such bad things to another (human) being without feeling the slightest bit of guilt. The dissociation would also explain why my Mum keeps denying that anything ever happened. Perhaps she has no memory of it, due to the (possible) dissociation.

Whatever it was, I now can say that I was terrified of my Mum, but back then I wasn't able to admit this. And even today I find it really hard to admit.

I have already mentioned that my Mum was very religious. This was probably the reason she found a job within the church. Even though it's hard for me to admit, she is really good at her job, which makes it all very complicated for me.
My Mum was kind, gentle and soft to all the people she worked with. She was there for them when they needed her. People from the parish constantly described her as a good and noble person, who always did the right thing (like some kind of angel).
But I knew a totally different woman, an unpredictable, aggressive tyrant, in which it was very difficult to see something good (like some kind of devil).

My Mum, for a very long time, had power over me. In some ways she still has.
For all the years that I was living at home I was her puppet. She pulled the strings and I moved the way she wanted me to. When I left home, I still visited my parents every weekend, when, again, I would become that puppet on a string. Even in my own apartment she continued to have power over me by harassing and threatening me with telephone calls, text messages, cards etc. So, in some way, she still had power over me even though I wasn't living with her anymore.

It didn't matter how hard I tried to create a certain distance and to live my own life. By visiting my parents every weekend I wasn't doing myself any favours. After every visit, I would have to start all over again.

One day, both of my parents came to visit me. This visit didn't turn out so well. I can't remember all the details anymore (and I'm glad about that). I do remember that I had to kick my Mum out of the house in a very negative manner.
From that moment onwards I decided to break contact with both of them. I wasn't able to fully do so, but it did mean that I wasn't going home anymore and no longer called, texted or wrote to them.

Yet the harm was already done. From that moment onwards I started to hear 'The Mother Voice'. This voice said the most horrible things in a very sweet tone. And as if this wasn't confusing enough, I also started to see an image of 'The Mother Voice' as well. I saw 'The Mother Voice' following me around all the time, or appearing right in front of me when I least expected it. She was following me everywhere and never gave me a break. She startled me all the time. She told me that I was the Devil and that I had to die. She told me that I should kill myself. It all seemed to boil down to the notion that I was evil and was to blame for all the suffering in the world.

Very often I struggled to distinguish certain things. I found it difficult to discern what was part of/belonged to my real life Mum, what belonged to 'The Mother Voice' and what belonged to 'The Mother Voice Image'. It really confused me and totally scared me.

Sometimes, people used to ask me what 'The Mother Voice Image' looked like. Did she look like my real life Mum or not? Because I didn't see my real life Mum for a very long time, I found that a difficult question to answer.
In the last couple of months I have seen my real life Mum and I think I can now say a full 'yes' to that question. 'The Mother Voice Image' definitely looks like my real life Mum, but the Mum from years and years ago, from the time when I was still living at home with her.
Yet to the question of whether this helps me to distinguish the real life Mum from 'The Mother Voice Image', I have to say 'no'. When

'The Mother Voice Image' appears, my fear will automatically take over. This prevents me from having a close look at 'The Mother Voice Image', to spot the difference so to speak. Fear does weird things to perception, that's for sure.

Every time I received a message from my parents, things went very wrong. 'The Mother Voice' became more active and most of the time 'The Mother Voice Image' would appear too.
I couldn't have received a clearer sign that contact with my real life Mum was not a good idea, but loyalty is a funny thing. Loyalty makes it incredibly difficult to do the thing you know is best for you: in my case, breaking all contact forever.

Over the past few years, I have been doing a lot better. I have minimised contact even more and that works out fine for me.
While I was writing this book, however, I was put to the test big time! Writing and telling my story is something I find really difficult and complicated. I've never wanted to harm anyone or to blame my parents. All I want is to explain that hearing voices is a 'cause and effect' thing and doesn't come out of the blue.
It's not my intention to say that it's my parents' fault, or that they are to blame. Yet the fact that things in our family and at our house were not as they were supposed to be is very clear. By now, I'm really convinced that if my parents had known better, had known a way to do things differently, they probably would have done so. But that's not the case, for whatever reason.

It took me a very long time to be able to look at things like this. It's still not always easy. Yet blaming my parents is not going to help me and it won't undo what has been done, so I try not to go down that road anymore. This doesn't mean, by the way, that I can forgive everything and forget it all.

During the writing of this book, I got some messages from my Mum that my Dad was really ill. From these messages it sounded as though my Dad was not going to make it much longer on this planet. And even though I have a very difficult relationship with my Mum, I do love my Dad very much. So this announcement about his health was something that really scared me.

'The Mother Voice' was immediately present and tried to convince me that it was my fault that my Dad was about to die. 'The Mother Voice Image' also appeared and added that she came back to finish what she didn't manage to finish before. This really confused me. In the past, my real life Mum made several attempts to kill both me and my Dad. So talking about 'finishing what she didn't manage to finish before' made me anxious and terrified. Both 'The Mother Voice' and 'The Mother Voice Image' made the threat that if I continued to write my book and went on to publish it, my Dad would have to pay the price for my actions. And I could add this to the list of 'evil deeds' together with the death of both my Granny and my dog.

I became really confused and wasn't able to write anymore. I had to fight really hard not to have a mental breakdown again, and I did succeed. I managed to get back on track. I did not have a breakdown and I picked up with the writing again.

If you were to ask me what 'The Mother Voice' and 'The Mother Voice Image' represent, I would have to honestly admit that this is one of the voices that I still can't look at or think about. My fear is too huge and gets in the way of having a good look at it. I can't promise that this will ever change; that I will have a closer look at it in the future. Right now, I don't really feel any necessity to look at it more closely. I know 'The Mother Voice' and 'The Mother Voice Image' can emerge, I know I will be scared again when this happens and I know that I have to figure out a way of dealing with this. As it currently stands, I can accept and live with the idea of not confronting this voice.

What I do know is that 'The Mother Voice' represents my terror and my fear of my real life Mum. I wasn't allowed to feel or express this fear, and didn't even know how to do so.

I also think that 'The Mother Voice' has a lot to do with my feelings of guilt. I feel responsible for, and guilty about, my dog's death and also my Granny's death. Somewhere in my brain the idea is lodged that if I had been sweeter, braver, or whatever, if I had done something, stepped up, I could have prevented my dog from being killed. If I had been sweeter, not such a pain in the ass, if I had needed less care, I might have prevented my Granny from getting cancer and dying.

Sure, I know I'm not really to blame for these things. But the fact that I know it does not automatically make me feel and experience my guilt any differently.

Besides all of this, I also feel incredibly guilty about all the suffering I caused my family by getting admitted to the child and adolescent psychiatric ward (and, later on, being treated within adult psychiatry). This is something 'The Mother Voice' likes to mention and (ab)use.

I know that these thoughts and feelings don't make any sense, and that it's kind of the world upside down. I know that I'm not to blame and that it was all the consequence of a really bad situation at home. But the fact that I know all of this does not change the way I feel about it.

The big theme or, more precisely, the big themes here are clear: feelings of fear and guilt.

The triggers for this voice and image have to do with things being unpredictable and unclear which makes me feel unsafe.

I'm pretty sure that I still have lots of work to do with this voice and everything she represents. There is still lots to go through. But as I said earlier, I'm not ready yet and I can't guarantee that I ever will be.

This is also the only voice where I can't say 100% confidently that I would not like her to go away. I think that if 'The Mother Voice' disappeared for good tomorrow, I would not miss her very much...

* dissociate: (very simple explanation) some kind of disconnection from the body and emotions, which makes it possible to cope with overwhelming emotions and situations, so you don't have to consciously experience them. Often, people who dissociate don't have any memory of what happened and might say they 'lost time'.

De Joachimstem
('The Joachim Voice')

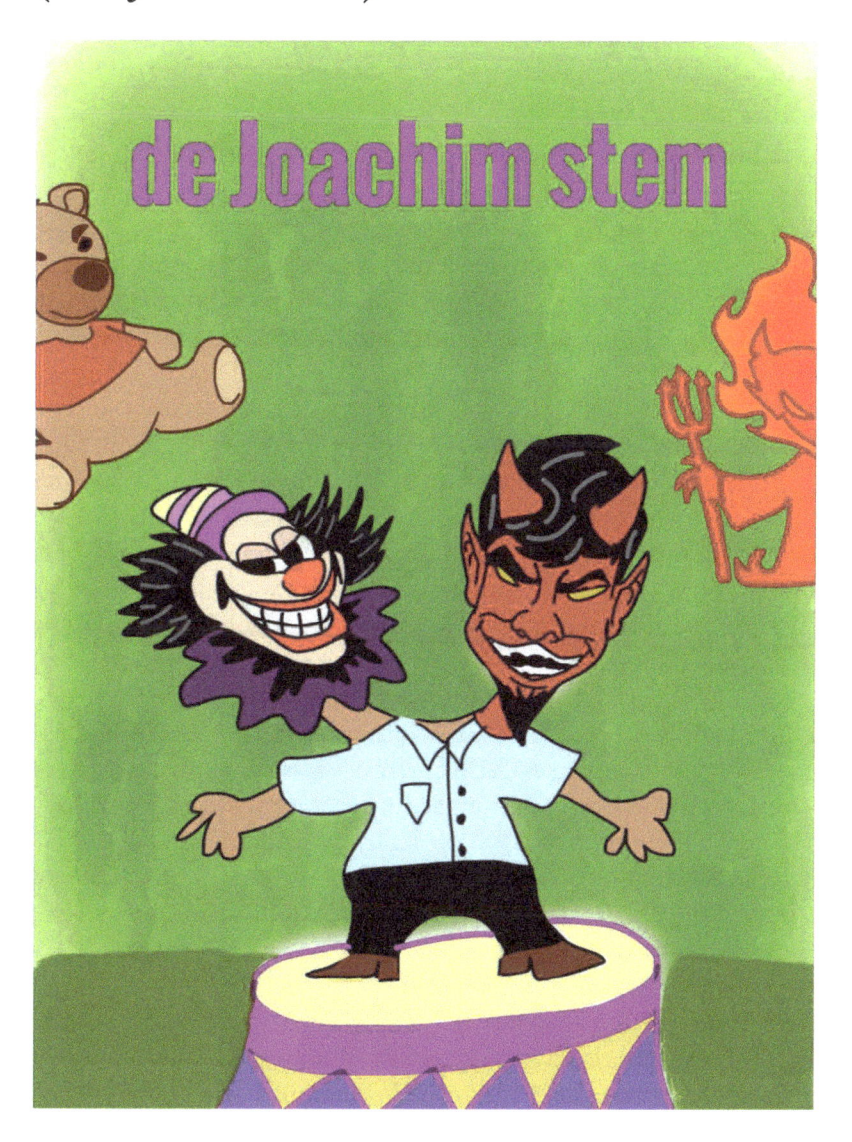

This voice is another one for which I can't remember exactly when it appeared for the first time. But that doesn't hinder me from telling you something about it.

In 2007 I was asked to be part of a team delivering workshops about coping with voices in a different way to the one being 'taught' in regular psychiatry. This really appealed to me. One of the reasons this appealed so much to me was that the method being spread via these workshops changed my own life entirely. I could even say that it saved my life. It is my wish that every voice hearer who is struggling with their voices can have access to this method and knowledge.

Another reason for doing the workshops was a bit less noble, and maybe even selfish: I love travelling and speaking other languages. These workshops were scheduled to take place in various countries other than my own. So, in my eyes, I would be able to do something useful in combination with something that I happen to find very pleasurable. So I decided to say 'yes' to this new challenge. But, as always, I immediately started to doubt myself over whether I would be 'good enough' to do this.

I also didn't know exactly what I was getting myself into. Within these workshops I was working together with two colleagues. Neither of them are Dutch and our common language is German, because that's the language all three of us have (at least) a basic knowledge of. We are quite an international crew, we all live in different countries, and we all have a different language as our mother tongue. A challenge in itself!

We are all very different types of people (and personalities). I am someone who needs clarity, predictability and structure. These things give me a sense of security, within which I can function.

One of my colleagues is called Joachim. And all of my above mentioned needs are not (at) all on his priority list. He has his own style of doing things and is able to cope with last minute things, changes and improvisations. These are not things I can cope with very well, especially not in a language other than my mother tongue. These differences would clash sometimes when we were together for our workshops.

Add a third colleague into the mix with her own needs, desires and style... and a potential script for a comedy of errors emerges.

Despite the fact that I really liked doing the work, it didn't go smoothly. I wasn't involved in these workshops from the beginning as my two colleagues were. They had already known each other for a long period of time when I joined the team and had a history together that I was unaware of, and wasn't a part of. It was very tricky for me and I felt very awkward a lot of the time. I felt misunderstood and unequal. My sixth sense told me that there was something going on, but I could not explain what it was that I sensed.

When we started working together I was mainly preoccupied with: "Am I doing well enough?", "Will they kick me out?", "Are they already searching for someone else, someone better than me?". All of these insecurities made me act in a way in which I was continuously trying to please Joachim.
Yet there was so much going on and so much happening that I didn't agree with. There were things that felt entirely wrong in my heart, yet I always kept quiet about them, just to keep the peace. I also kept my mouth shut because I was afraid of being sent away.
I rarely spoke my mind. But when the tension inside got to boiling point, I usually failed to make it to the end of the workshop, instead leaving earlier. I left in anger, without telling anyone what was bothering me. (In defence of myself I want to say that I sometimes

really tried to speak my mind, but found it very complicated to do so as I didn't feel heard or listened to).

At some point during or after one of our workshops, I started to hear 'De Joachimstem': 'The Joachim Voice'. His tone of voice sounded exactly like the real life Joachim. They were hard to differentiate from one another.
'The Joachim Voice' kept changing languages, just like the real life Joachim, and just as I sometimes used to do during the workshops. 'The Joachim Voice' speaks both English and German and sometimes even Dutch, which is something the real life Joachim can't do. So this is something that differentiates them.

'The Joachim Voice' would say a lot of mean things, just like my Mum would do. On the other hand, he could also say very nice things, but in a very mocking kind of tone. However, I struggled to know how to interpret the things 'The Joachim Voice' would say. This made me feel totally confused a lot of the time.
It was during these moments of confusion that I would start to lose it as I couldn't work out if what had just been said was a genuine comment or if it was a joke. This was very unclear to me.

As if this wasn't confusing enough, I would sometimes also see a 'Joachim Image' as well. Sometimes during the workshops there could be two versions of Joachim standing next to one another (the real life Joachim and 'The Joachim Image'). At some times I didn't have any idea which one was the real life Joachim.

Maybe you can imagine that it's very confusing and fear-provoking to see the real life Joachim and 'The Joachim Image' standing next to each other, talking at the same time. The confusion would be heightened when the real life Joachim would say something entirely in opposition to 'The Joachim Image'. Just like it is with 'The Mother Voice' and/or 'The Mother Voice Image', I could no longer tell where the real life person, the voice and the image started and ended when this happened. In short, this led to a lot of confusing situations in my head which I didn't always know how to solve.

This didn't only happen during workshops. It was also the case that when I was at home in my apartment I would start to hear 'The Joachim Voice'. This mostly happened at those times when we had recent contact about an upcoming workshop over the phone or Skype and when some of the information wasn't entirely clear to me, or I disagreed and felt unable (or hadn't even tried at all) to speak my mind. It could also happen when I was feeling unsafe or when things occurred that felt entirely unpredictable.

As my colleague lived in the United Kingdom at that time, you could be forgiven for thinking that it should have been a piece of cake for me to know that, as soon as 'The Joachim Image' appeared in my apartment, something was wrong. And, yes, I have to admit that this should have been clear to me, but in those moments I was so scared and confused that logical thinking ceased to be one of my strengths.

When this first started to happen, I tried to check if my colleague was indeed in my apartment. So I called his UK number. As soon as he answered his phone, things were simple. This was until 'The Mother Voice' whispered in my ear that, in this era of mobile phone connections, you can never be sure of anything. And in this case, on this topic, she had a point.

So I started to check where the real-life Joachim was via his landline phone. If he picked up, I knew for certain that what I saw and heard (in my apartment) were not actually happening, and I felt relieved for a while. Yet this wasn't always enough proof as 'The Mother Voice' also whispered in my ear that there was a possibility of forwarding messages to different numbers.

In everyday life, between the workshops, my colleague and I had contact on a regular basis. Also in real life, as a person, my colleague was, and continues to be, a big mystery to me. I still can't always interpret what he means. Is it a joke, or is he being serious? This makes him a person who feels rather unpredictable and unsafe to me. The voice and the image, therefore, match strongly with how I experience my colleague in real life.

My colleague has had to deal with my voices every now and again, without me knowing about this (in other words, when I had dissociated). Lesley, especially, would come out as she really likes my colleague. She has never been able to remember or pronounce his name, so she decided to call him 'Bear'. He earned this name because he tells her a story about a bear over and over again if he wants me, Mick, to return and take charge again. Lesley doesn't understand what he is telling her as the story is in German and Lesley can only understand spoken Dutch and Dutch sign language. Yet she does know it's about a Mummy bear, a Daddy bear and baby bear. She thinks that 'Bear' (my colleague) sounds really funny when he tells this story. His story is a big hit with Lesley, but he has hardly ever succeeded in his goal (of getting Mick back in charge) by telling it.

Lesley thinks that 'Bear' is talking in a funny way. She is convinced that 'Bear' can speak Dutch as she heard him do so on a couple of occasions. I can't explain to her that 'Bear', when speaking to his Mum and Dad, is speaking a dialect that sounds similar to Dutch, so she can understand him then. She cannot understand that 'Bear' is 'not smart enough' to understand her. Even though Lesley still doesn't entirely believe me, she now also uses her hands (sign language) when talking to him, although not very successfully by the way!

If I were to give you a summary, I would say that I still don't really know what the role of this voice is in my life. It can be pretty complicated at times. I do know for sure that there is a connection with things being unclear and unpredictable, and with not knowing where I stand.

I can't say for sure if I would mind if this voice left. I think it would make life much easier and less confusing if he wasn't there. Yet I can also live with this voice being around, as it reminds me constantly of the need to speak my mind when I don't like something or am required to stand up for myself.

De Dirkstem
('The Dirk Voice')

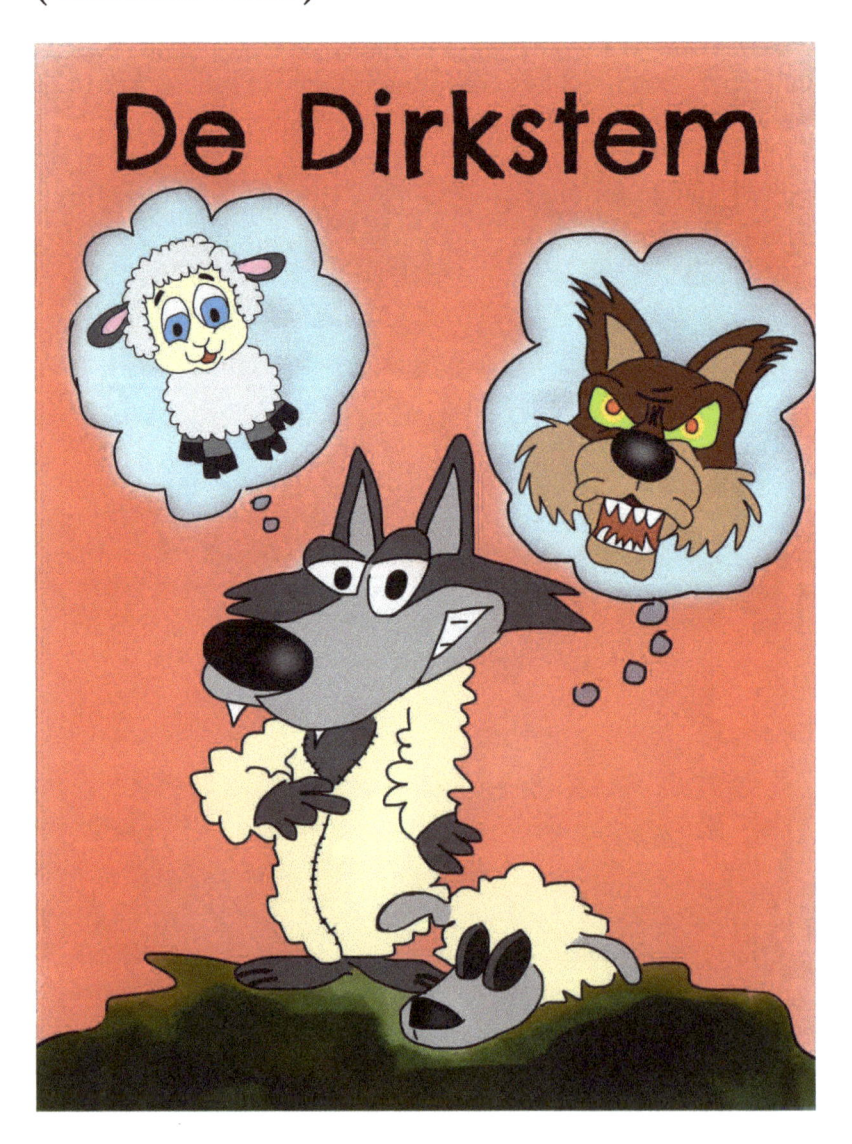

'The Dirk Voice' is a complicated voice to describe in several ways. I don't exactly know when he appeared for the first time and I also don't have a well thought-out explanation for him. But I will try to tell you something about him.

When I ended up in psychiatry as an adult, I wasn't doing very well. I had kind of unlearned how to talk (which had never been a hobby of mine). I was utterly convinced that it would not matter if I talked or not as no one would believe me anyway. So I didn't even try to speak. I compensated for my lack of words (unconsciously) with very strong body language. This was so strong that I hardly had any need of words to express my thoughts or feelings. People could (literally) see what I was thinking or how I felt.

During this time I was assigned a therapist who I could talk to on a weekly basis. In addition to him I was given a crisis manager whose job it was to deal with the moments of crisis in my life. The therapist and I did not really 'click'. He needed to work via a strict protocol (due to our sessions being part of a scientific research project) and wasn't allowed to ask me any questions. This made it difficult to form a connection with him. Everything that was spoken about had to come from me. This was not a smart set-up as being silent was one of the qualities no one could beat me at. So I would simply not say anything at all.

When I showed up at my crisis manager's desk, he did ask me questions. This made it at least a bit easier to speak about what was going on inside of me. He may not have noticed that he made it easier for me as he still had to work his arse off to get me to speak.
In those days I was being very much bothered by the voices and didn't know how to cope with them at all. So my life became a series of crisis moments. I hadn't yet told anyone about the voices, so no one knew what was going on inside of me. I didn't tell them as I was afraid of getting a diagnosis of schizophrenia, of being locked up, and

of being pumped with medication. This was what I had been taught about hearing voices during my psychology course. I was taught that the lives of people with a diagnosis of schizophrenia could only go downhill. I had learnt that the only treatment consisted of taking strong medication for the rest of your life. This was not how I wanted to see my life playing out. So I kept my mouth shut about what I was hearing.

Eventually, things went wrong and I ended up in a crisis centre. At this point the voices kind of took over my life. I was so afraid of what they were saying that I did almost everything I could to keep them satisfied. By doing so I ended up in the crisis centre, but I still didn't tell anyone about the voices.

It got to the point where staff no longer had a clue about how to deal with me, so they called the crisis manager. He came to the centre on his bike after working hours. He lit a cigarette in the centre's living room. That was against the rules, so I kind of liked what I saw: a professional who didn't obey the rules!

This man was the first person to whom I admitted I was hearing voices and who didn't freak out over it. He just started asking me questions about them. And, strangely enough, I found it a very nice experience not to have to keep my secret (or, at least, one of my many secrets) hidden anymore. I found it even more strange that, at the end of our conversation, he sent me home instead of sectioning me (which is what the plan of the staff had been). He sent me home with a promise that we would work on a 'solution' for the voices.

The crisis manager's name was Dirk. In relation to the voices, he put me right back on track. He taught me to explore the voices and how to see connections between the voices and my life history. He even taught me how to talk to, and really listen to, the voices. This is something I'm still grateful for every day, as it gave me back my life.

When I first walked into his office, I didn't trust anyone or anything. As I have written before, Dirk had to work his arse off to establish the slightest form of a connection with me.

Over the years, I started to see Dirk as a kind of 'loving Dad' who never got angry, who didn't give me any boundaries, but who led me gently but firmly back on track when I crossed the invisible boundaries (as there certainly were boundaries!) without me even noticing that he was doing so.
This continued for years and he became the most important person in my life. If something happened, good or bad, he was the first person who came to my mind to share it with. Whereas my friends would call their parents or siblings, the only person who came to my mind was my 'replacement parent'. So I would contact Dirk.

But after years of being the 'loving Dad', the image started to crack a bit. He became less patient. He even got angry every now and again and would really show his anger. At the same time, I had become more mature and more empowered. If I had any thoughts on a topic I would say so, whether it was welcome or not. So these two things clashed more and more and we ended up having some seriously heated discussions.
My explanation for all of this, for a very long time, was to see it as some kind of parenting situation. When I first entered Dirk's office, I was a small, scared, abandoned child who wasn't able to trust anyone or anything. He was there as a 'loving Dad', took me under his wing, and made it possible for me to first trust him and, later on, to trust others as well. But babies and small children grow up. So when the heated discussions and arguments started, I saw myself as a teenager rebelling against the 'loving Dad'. This drove Dirk insane from time to time and made him angry.

These 'fights' or arguments triggered a lot of uncertainty in me. Out of the blue (at least in my experience) there were suddenly boundaries and a change in Dirk's behaviour. I didn't understand why and couldn't cope with the perceived changes very well. I didn't like it one bit. It made me scared of Dirk and I came to feel very uncertain of him.

Dirk became an unpredictable, and therefore unsafe, factor in my life. I find it very difficult to admit that he reminded me of my Mum during that time. This made it very difficult to unite the 'old' Dirk with this 'new' Dirk.

I think that might have been the point when I started to hear 'The Dirk Voice'. This voice tends to sound really calm and relaxed, like the 'loving Dad' version of Dirk, but it also says some of the same kinds of things my Mum used to say. 'The Dirk Voice' bashes me, humiliates me, and calls me names.
'The Dirk Voice' will say, in a friendly, calm voice, that I'm useless and will never amount to anything. It tells me that I'm not worthy of the oxygen on this Earth and that the world would be a better place without me.

Because 'The Dirk Voice's' tone of voice is exactly the same as the real life Dirk, it is sometimes complicated to tell them apart. 'The Dirk Voice' made my fear of Dirk grow to the point where working with him was no longer an option.

In 2014, after having worked together for fifteen years, I finally untied the knot. By this time, Dirk had become so unpredictable and, therefore, unsafe to me that I hardly dared to say or share anything with him without having the fear of starting another heated discussion or argument. It was no longer possible to work together. After a lot of thinking and the copious shedding of tears I decided to ask for another professional.

This was one of the hardest decisions of my life but, at the same time, it might have been one of the best decisions. Only when the relationship between Dirk and myself got worse did I begin to realise how dependent on Dirk I had become. This was something I would never want to experience again! Thanks to this realisation, I think I became a lot stronger in making (and standing by) my decisions.

What I love about 'The Dirk Voice' is that, after the decision to ask for someone else, he calmed down a lot. 'The Dirk Voice' is not gone but is only present when I'm still struggling with 'Dirk related issues' or when 'De Heilige Drie Eenheid' ('The Holy Trinity', which you will read more about in the next chapter) comes together. But this doesn't happen quite as much anymore either.

'The Holy Trinity'

Besides the fact that voices can act on their own, there can also be some cooperation between them. I would like to describe one of these cooperatives. I sometimes refer to them as 'The Holy Trinity'. This cooperative contains 'De Moederstem' ('The Mother Voice'), 'De Joachimstem' ('The Joachim Voice') and 'De Dirkstem' ('The Dirk Voice').

These three voices (often) work together and this doesn't make things exactly easy for me. At the same time it makes absolute sense to me now and I find it very logical. But this has not always been the case.

I have already told you about my time working abroad and delivering workshops on making sense of hearing voices. During these workshops things would spin out of control for me quite often. I got angry and would walk away when things seemed unclear. These three voices played a huge part in this. I will try to explain how they did so.

At those times when things started to get difficult for me during these workshops, I would start to hear 'The Joachim Voice'. This usually happened when things were being said that I didn't agree with, which made me angry or sad. Nowadays I'm a bit better at it but, for a very long time, I didn't dare to speak my mind or object to the things I disagreed with. Keeping silent increased the anger and sadness. By not speaking my mind and bottling up these negative emotions, I felt worse and worse. If it got too bad, 'The Joachim Image' would appear in addition to 'The Joachim Voice'. This marked the start of complete confusion for me.

This situation makes me very paranoid as there are three versions of Joachim I have to deal with. I no longer have any idea of which version I should pay attention to in order to get the 'correct information'. Even if I were able to understand which of these three is my colleague, I find him very unpredictable as a person as well.

After all these years, I still can't always tell when he is joking and when he's being serious. So I'm never sure how to assess what has been said, which makes me feel very insecure.
In these kinds of situations it feels as though the real-life Joachim is trying to fool me. I then try to fit in everything he says or does into this theory of his foolery. This makes me feel paranoid and I start to question everything he says or does, even the most innocent of words or gestures.

In moments like this, I feel very bad about myself. I feel entirely worthless, unfit as a person and also inferior.

These feelings are the cue for 'The Mother Voice' to get involved in the situation. This can be with, or without 'The Mother Voice Image'. She will do everything to perpetuate these bad feelings about myself and, if possible, she will try to make things even worse. She belittles me, criticises me and repeats how worthless and bad I really am. She tells me that I should not have been born at all, that I'm not worth the oxygen on the Earth and that I should kill myself as the whole world and everyone in it would be better off without me.

If I resist long enough and act as though I don't care and that her words do not hurt me (but of course, they do!), she will always add the sentence: "And you know it is true, Dirk says so too."

This is the cue for 'The Dirk Voice' to butt into the conversation and start being negative. This makes it impossible for me to figure out who or what to believe. So I start to get scared. The environment becomes a frightening place, as nothing and no one seems to be what or who they really are. There is only one thing I want in these moments: to run away from this unclear, unsafe space to my safe apartment back home!

This is what kept happening during these workshops.

The weird part is that, as soon as these three voices (and images) start to work together, the language they all communicate in changes to Dutch. If I would only be able to think rational thoughts at these times, this would be a sign for me that something was not quite right as my colleague can't speak any Dutch. But in moments like this, even after all these years, I can't think rationally about anything in these moments as I'm so overwhelmed by my emotions. The only thing I can think of is to get my stuff and jump on a train back home, as soon as possible.

Nowadays, this doesn't happen much. My explanation for this is that I try to speak my mind more and more. I try to not let all the tension and annoyance get to me and I make sure it doesn't reach the point when it will somehow explode. I make sure that I will be heard, that I say what needs to be said, even when it's not so easy to do! I don't do and say anything anymore that I don't agree with and I think this is the reason the tension and annoyance don't get to boiling point anymore.

By now, I have also learned to count to a hundred before replying or reacting to anything. More and more regularly, I choose to let things go as they are not worth my energy or the discussion.
This might sound contradictory to what I said before about speaking my mind but, in my opinion, it isn't. For me, the difference is in the fact that I now consciously choose if I want to expend my energy on something or not. I now choose if it's worth it to do so, or not. And I come to the conclusion, more and more, that it's simply not worth it.

What also helps quite a bit is that, without feeling guilty, I sometimes deliberately switch off my brain so I literally cannot hear the conversations (often monologues). I still don't find this very polite of me and I prefer not to do it, but I know that I sometimes have to this in order to protect myself. Since I have been allowing myself to do this, without feeling too guilty, I'm doing much better and 'The Holy

Trinity' is not doing so well as they don't have so much power over me anymore.

At the start of this chapter, I wrote that it is now logical and makes sense to me that these voices sometimes work together.

In the separate chapters about them, I told you about how these voices remind me, or make me think of, people that I know in real life. All of these real life people are very complicated to me. With all three of them I don't have a clue about how to assess them. This makes them really unpredictable and, as I have said (many times) before, unpredictable means unsafe to me. And unsafe feelings or circumstances make me feel really insecure.

'The Holy Trinity' comes at those times when I already feel insecure about myself and when the situation I'm in is not safe enough to allow me to be myself. In my opinion, they are a magnification. It would also be correct to say that they are a mirror: some kind of shaving mirror where one side shows true proportions and the other side magnifies the image. They show me how insecure I feel about something in a magnified way.

Today, 'The Holy Trinity' are not around too often and definitely not in such an amount that causes me to run off. But I certainly struggled with this for a long time and it took me even longer to see the similarities in these three voices.

By now, I'm convinced that when someone hears voices from people they know in real life this can lead to extra confusion and paranoia. I also believe that this can sometimes lead to difficult and even dangerous situations.

Nevertheless, I'm very grateful that 'The Holy Trinity' made things very difficult for me for a while and, from time to time, made it impossible for me to function. I did learn a lot from this. By making it impossible to function within something I actually really liked (doing the workshops) it created the necessity to find different ways of coping with the situation. And I'm not entirely sure that I would have started looking for these other ways if the voices had not have given me such a hard time.

So, even though it was very challenging at some times, it was definitely worth the struggle!

Muziek
(Music)

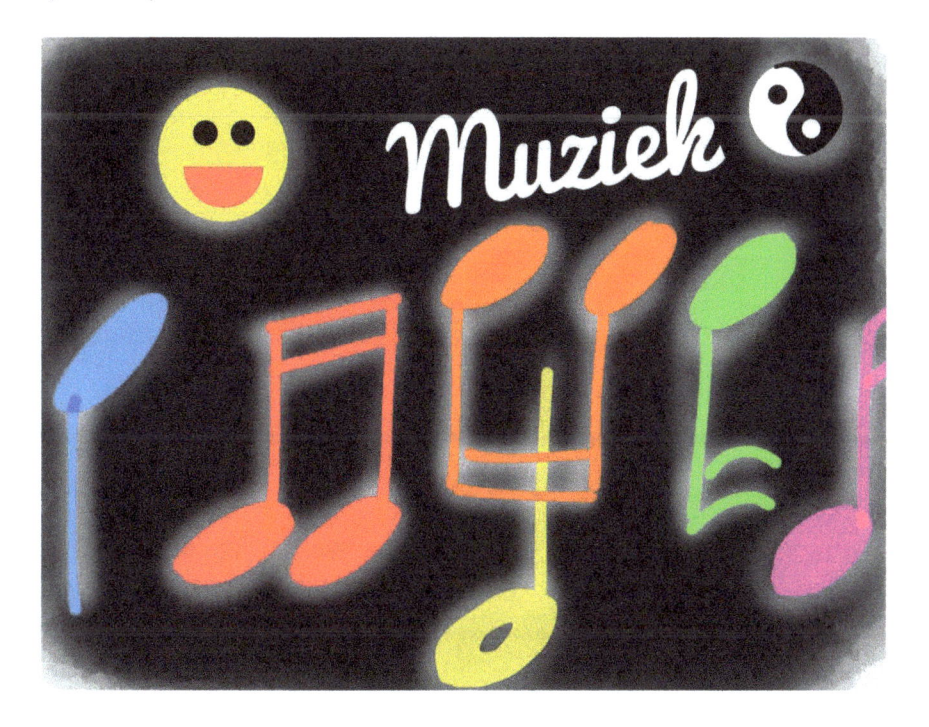

Last but not least there is one more voice I want to tell you something about. To me it's the 'newest voice'.

In 2013 I decided to go back to Australia. My first visit was in 2008. Although I really enjoyed that trip, I also was afraid of everything that moved or didn't move. I did see a lot of the country during that first trip, but I also didn't see a lot of the country. And because the World Hearing Voices Conference, just as in 2008, was going to take place in Australia that year, I decided to go there again. And this time I would stay as long as my Visa would permit it.
And so I did. I flew to the other side of the world on my own. I started my journey quite a while before the conference started and

also stayed quite a while after the conference finished. I planned to stay for a total of three months and in these months I was about to make some of my dreams come true.

One of these dreams was celebrating Christmas on Bondi Beach. But my biggest dream was to see the fireworks on the Sydney Harbour Bridge on New Year's Eve. And to top all of these dreams off, I wanted to have the 'longest birthday ever', which basically meant flying back home on my birthday. To me these three things were really important.

If you really knew me, you would know that I don't like 'unexpected things'. I get anxious when I don't know what is going to happen or if things don't go according to (my) plan. These kind of 'little things' can ruin my (not very strong) balance.
Because of this, my trip to Australia was a huge challenge for me. I did arrange some details beforehand, but most of my trip I didn't plan at all and I was about to see what would happen. And thinking of this, I got really nervous! But at the same time it felt like this was exactly the way I wanted to do things.

During my life I have noticed that I need literal distance from my home country to make important decisions, as this gives me time and space to think about stuff. This trip I had some things I really needed to think about.

My time in Australia was amazing and I really loved being there! I felt free in several ways. Australia is a beautiful country and I loved being outdoors most of the time, in contrast to the Netherlands where I spend most of my time inside my home.
Whereas I find it difficult at home to look people in the eye, to talk to them or to arrange things, while I was in Australia I did these things almost automatically. A different language can cause miracles to happen inside of me: it gives me distance from myself.

Possibly the biggest difference between Australia and the Netherlands is that, at home, I can't stop thinking. And thinking often morphs very easily into worrying so I seldom feel calm and relaxed a home.

During those three months I was travelling through Australia, I felt an inner peace I had never felt before. I felt completely happy! Utterly calm, free of worries, totally Zen.

One day, I was sitting in a very quiet place, eating dinner and watching the sunset. There were no people or houses nearby. And while I was watching the sunset and thinking about how happy and calm I felt, I started to hear music.

I heard soft, gentle classical music. Very pleasant to listen to. I'm not a huge lover of classical music and, until a couple of years before, I had never listened to this kind of music. So it felt kind of special in and of itself. I thought that the music must be coming from somewhere else, maybe one of the business accommodations behind me. So I didn't really give it my full attention.

One day I woke up in the middle of nowhere. It was really early and I decided to go for a hike. It was really calm and quiet inside my head: no thoughts, no voices, entirely quiet.
It was, in fact, so quiet, that for the first time in my life, I could hear the buzzing of the flies (and for those people who have ever been to Australia, there are many flies over there so the sound can be quite loud). This silence and hearing a simple sound like the buzzing of the flies made me the happiest human being on Earth.

In that moment I started to hear classical music again! And this time I was really sure it could not be coming from a house nearby, as there were no houses at all. I also was quite sure that the kangaroos and wallabies had not spontaneously decided to start an orchestra. So there couldn't be any other explanation: this music was inside my head, just playing for me.

There were more moments when I heard the music. All of these times were moments when I felt totally relaxed and Zen. Moments when I felt completely happy.

In Australia I felt relaxed, I could enjoy things, I was happy and I was worry-free for three months.

As soon as I got on the plane to return home, on my birthday, the worrying immediately returned. Apparently I wasn't able to hold on to this feeling of happiness.
As soon as I got home and tried to start living my life again, there were some brief moments when I could feel relaxed, sometimes even very happy. I was really surprised to find out that, during these moments, I would hear the classical music again.

To me this voice/sound is a symbol of the moments when I feel relaxed, calm, Zen and happy. So I'm really happy with this voice and don't want it to go away!

Epilogue

That's it: I have finished my book.

There is so much more to tell you about my voices, but I think I have covered the most important things I wanted to say for now.

Writing this book was quite a process. I discovered a lot of things about myself that I, deep down, already knew but would rather not have known about myself. It is a bit similar to the journey I have been on with my voices.

For example, at some point I discovered that I find it really difficult to ask other people for help. I knew very well what it is that I wanted and how I envisaged things as being with this book. I had an exact image in my head of how it should turn out. I also knew that I would get upset as soon as other people started to help me, as they would mess up the image I had inside my head. I don't like changes. This made it really complicated to ask people for help.

At the same time, I also knew there would come a point in publishing the book when I needed to ask for help. I know very well that I have limitations in what I can do and handle. If I look into something and there is too much information, I can't process it all. I get very angry with myself and become very upset. I become so frustrated that I am liable to throw it all aside and to quit. This is one of the reasons this book has not seen the daylight much sooner.

Looking into the 'how', 'what' and 'where' of publishing this book brought up so much more than I ever dreamed possible. It felt like an insurmountable hurdle and my plan of publishing a book was regularly put on hold. So, this time, I decided to write the damn book first and to worry about whether or not to publish it and how later.

Even though I knew this was going to be a big hurdle for me, and knew that I would need help with this (and also knew who I wanted this help from), it didn't make it any easier to ask for and accept help. The fact that I'm allowed to take up time and space, am allowed to ask for help and am worthy of accepting help from others are definitely some issues to work on over the coming years.

Even though I went through all of the publishing information and asking for help while writing the original Dutch version. It didn't make these things any easier when it came to asking for help with the English translation, nor with getting the translated version published. It was just as difficult as it was the first time round with the Dutch version!

I discovered that writing a book was a very fun and educational thing to do for me, but it also triggered a lot.
For example: the fact that I can no longer remember when all the voices first appeared, and in which circumstances, frustrated me enormously! How was it possible not to know such important information anymore?!?

Another issue was that I started to read old documents and files about what I (or the voices) said back then about them and their presence. A lot of the time I could not remember what was written down about that time and sometimes it even contradicted how I (and the voices themselves) think about the voices now. This was really difficult as both things, the not remembering and the contradictions, made me feel like I was being deceitful at times.

However, it also made it clear to me that I'm only human and human beings are a work in progress. So am I. My voices and the journey we have taken together are no exception to this. It's all a work in progress.

Writing also pointed out very clearly to me that I'm not there yet. There is still a lot to discover, to learn and also to process. The writing of this book triggered a lot. Many memories that I have not at all, or hardly, talked about yet.

At some point this almost pushed me over the edge because the past, the present, and the 'voice world' started to get mixed up again. But I made it! Even during the translation of this book, at some moments it still made me emotionally very wobbly. At these times, I had to put the text aside for a while to be able to re-find my balance.

I might not be there yet. I'm not even sure where I have to go in order to be 'there'. I'm not even sure if I ever will get 'there'. The only thing I know for certain is that I'm on my way. And that's more than enough.

It's all in my head! All fifteen of the voices are travelling along with me, every day, every hour, every second. For now, my mission is accomplished. I have finished my book. I hope this book has given you some insight into how voices can come into existence, how they can influence us and how they can sometimes even take over our lives. It is my hope that it has also shown you that there can be light at the end of the tunnel if you are able to find a way to cope with them.

I hope I was able to make it clear to you that while it all might be in my head, that doesn't mean it's any less real. My voices are real, each and every one of them. They are there, they exist, and they are undeniable!

Thank you for taking the time to read my book,

Mick

Acknowledgements:

Writing a chapter with acknowledgements…

After having written an entire book, this might be the most difficult part to write. Not the writing in itself (I have some practice in writing by now!) but acknowledgements are a scary thing to write.

In the acknowledgements chapter, the author, as the word suggests, acknowledges people who, in some way, shape or form, helped them to create this book. But what if, by accident, they forget to mention someone? Isn't that going to hurt people, even though that is not what they intended to do?
Of course I can tell myself that I don't have any power over how other people feel and that this would be their own problem, but I'm not very good at thinking like this. I know from experience what it is like to be forgotten and that's a horrible feeling.

So, I would love to suffice with the announcement that I'm very grateful for everyone who, in some way, shape or form, contributed to the existence of both the original and translated version of my book. A huge thank you from the bottom of my heart.

But I can't (and don't want to) avoid mentioning and thanking some people by name in no particular order.

So, here I go…

First of all, a huge thank you to Rich and Yvonne. Without your invitation (or, shall I call it, challenge?) and support, this book would not have been written. Thank you for giving me a chance and for believing in me.

Also a huge thank you to my fantastic buddy Martha. I want to thank you for being my cheerleader, for reading through the manuscript with me, for asking me questions, for your encouraging words, for your supportive postcards, for having the patience of an angel, and for your beautiful smile on Skype. It made me feel as though the sun were appearing on my screen!

A big thank you also to David and Diana, two angels who, with lots of love and patience, made time in their busy schedules to help me with the things that were so difficult for me. Thank you for helping me to de-clutter the chaos in my head, and for preparing me for Copyright issues so I would not entirely freak out during the process. Thank you for your companionship and for the lunches and tea we had together. Thank you for lending me your ears and for all the hugs to celebrate the many small and big steps along the way. And, last but not least, thank you for being you!

And, of course, I want to say thank you to Dirk. I know I'm not allowed to glorify you, but I'm so grateful for you that I could write an entirely new book about it (don't worry Dirk, I won't). For now, I will reduce it by just thanking you for writing your kind words at the start of this book and for all the years you believed in me, even during the times I could not believe in myself. And thank you for all the patience you have had with me.

Emilia, I also want to thank you for so much more than I can tell. You gave me words for the things I wasn't able to say. You kept believing in me, even though I gave you a hard time every now and again. Thank you for opening my eyes and showing me that the things that have happened to me were really bad. I think you still haven't grasped the enormity of the gift you gave to me by showing me this.

Thanks also to my psychologist, who willingly listened to my stories about the writing process, and all the ups and downs that came along with it, over and over again. Thank you Pom, you rock!

Thank you Joachim for your support and for being part of this journey of making sense of my experiences. Thank you especially for your patience with both myself and the voices. We are aware of the fact that we did not always give you an easy time.

Also a thank you to the team of The Choir Press and especially Miles for helping out with the cover design and everything else.

And then, last but definitely not least, there is the amazing Nicole Schnackenberg, who helped me to 'Englify' my translation and supported me through the 'wood of information' related to publishing this English version. Thank you for all the time you spent on correcting my translation and for so much more. Thank you for all the lovely conversations, for the tea, for the long walks along the beach, for your hospitality, and for your lovely hugs. Thank you for your support, your love, and for so much more! Thank you for being you! Thank you for being my friend!

Thank you to everyone around me who cares about me and keeps believing in me, even when I'm giving you all a hard time.

Thanks to all the readers for buying and reading this book. I hope it gave you some new insights and maybe an occasional smile.

Last but not least I want to thank my voices. Thank you for trying to help me, all in your own unique ways. Thanks for letting me illustrate you, and for letting me ask you a million questions (and still not understanding what you meant). This way, you have helped me to tell your (and, therefore, my) story. Without you guys, this book would not have been written in the first place.

Thank you all. I feel so grateful!

Mick, December 2017